MALARIA

MALARIA

A *layman's* guide

MARTINE MAUREL

SOUTHERN
BOOK PUBLISHERS

Dedication

For my beloved son, Nicholas, who before his third year of life grappled five times with the malaria monster and lived to tell the tale.

ISBN 1 86812 534 3
First edition, first impression 1994
First edition, second impression 1996
Published by Southern Book Publishers (Pty) Ltd
PO Box 3103, Halfway House, 1685
South Africa

Set in 10 on 12 point Palatino
by P. de Zeeuw
Printed and bound by National Book Printers,
Drukkery Street, Goodwood, Western Cape

Disclaimer

Should the reader suspect a malaria condition in himself or any
other person, he should make every effort to consult a medical doctor for professional assistance before either treating or not treating
himself or that other person. No responsibility will be taken by the
author or publisher for any illness or other inconvenience that may
result from information given in this book.

Acknowledgements

I wish to thank Dr Terry Taylor of the Malaria Project Unit at Queen Elizabeth Hospital in Blantyre, Malawi; Dr Eddie Hall, formerly of the Intensive Care Unit at the same hospital and Dr Gilbert Burnham of Johns Hopkins University, Baltimore, USA for their invaluable help and encouragement. Grateful thanks also to my commissioning editor, Louise Grantham, for her unwavering faith in the project and to my father, Colin Slater, for his commitment and dedication in guiding the book through to completion.

Preface

Most doctors in malaria-endemic countries know about malaria. In contrast, doctors in non-malarious countries know very little about it, perhaps understandably. Neither do most ordinary, non-medical people who are likely to come into contact with malaria. This book is for them.

Instead of trying to find out the hard way, through dribs and drabs of information passed on from friend to friend, doctor to patient, and possibly learnt through bitter frightening experience, your time will be saved if you read this book and keep it as a handy companion on your travels. The knowledge imparted here is readily digestible and not couched in swathes of unintelligible medical jargon.

If you are likely to be placed in a position similar to one of the following scenarios, you will need this book:

- ✧ You are the mother of an infant and are visiting a tropical country. Your child has a high fever and you suspect malaria. You are three hours away from a doctor by road and it is midnight. The phone doesn't work or the doctor is not in. What action should you take?
- ✧ You are a business traveller and have recently returned to South Africa from a trip to Malawi. Although you took your prophylactics as directed for the duration of your trip and for the recommended period afterwards, it is now four weeks since you have returned home and your bones and joints ache, you have a headache, it is freezing midwinter and your doctor tells you you have a dose of flu. You suspect malaria. How can you prove to him that he is wrong?
- ✧ You are an expatriate or aid worker living in Kenya, where you are exposed to much expatriate folklore about malaria. You will be living there for three years. Should you take prophylaxis?
- ✧ You return to South Africa after a holiday in Zimbabwe. You develop the classic symptoms of malaria but the blood test proves to be negative. Your doctor refuses to treat on the basis

of a negative blood test. Time is critical. Should you urge him to treat you anyway?

This book was born out of a baptism of fire. From the age of seven months, my second child suffered five bouts of malaria in one year. The long, lonely hours I spent deep in the night wondering whether he was going to live or die, and knowing that I had conflicting advice from whichever doctor I turned to, prompted me to write this book. Instead of being a mysterious disease to ordinary people who are its victims, malaria needs to be brought out in the open and become understandable.

As the staff of the Malaria Control Unit of the WHO (World Health Organization) point out: "Ultimately, only people who are well informed [about malaria] hold the key to a malaria-free future".

Contents

Other measures to take to help minimise the effects of malaria; Drug administration and absorption

Introduction

Malaria kills two people every minute. Each year, more than one million people die from malaria and over 100 million suffer potentially fatal cases. The disease threatens 2 220 million people, almost half of the world's population.

African countries south of the Sahara desert account for 80 per cent of all clinical cases and nearly 80 per cent of deaths caused by malaria. Children are most vulnerable to this major killer. In rural, tropical African areas, one in 20 children die from malaria before they reach the age of five years.

Despite a ray of hope in the 1960s, when chemical spraying with DDT seemed to control the malaria menace and before it was realised that DDT itself was a killer, reported cases and deaths caused by malaria are rising. The WHO has recently changed its focus from one of eradication to one of control.

The WHO was so alarmed by the rise in malaria incidence that it called a special Ministerial Conference concentrating only on malaria which was held in Amsterdam in 1992.

A number of strategies have been outlined by the WHO to attempt to achieve this control. One of these strategies includes prompt diagnosis and treatment and this can only be achieved through knowledge and information being available to the doctor and the patient so that each may recognise malaria in good time.

How to use this book

Note that there is a certain amount of duplication between chapters. Please bear with the author as far as this is concerned as it is intended to simplify the answering of questions for the reader, thus making the book user-friendly. Where pertinent, cross-references to other chapters have been made.

The book is not intended to be read from cover to cover. Rather it should be used as a reference book: to explain something your doctor mentioned but did not clarify; to answer your urgent questions when a life is at stake and you have no access to medical knowledge; to inform you exactly what the parameters of malaria are, so that it is no longer an awesome, unintelligible disease that is largely speculated about.

1. What is malaria?

Malaria is a disease caused by four species of parasite that are carried from person to person by a mosquito and transmitted by the bite of an infected female Anopheles mosquito.

The disease causes the blood to lose its oxygen-carrying capacity by bursting the blood cells that are infected. The debris arising from this causes a clogging of the arteries to the kidneys, lungs and brain which in the long term can be fatal.

If left untreated, malaria caused by one of the four parasites, *Plasmodium falciparum*, results in death which can occur in a relatively short space of time, from just over 12 hours to a few days.

Malaria caused by the other three parasites *Plasmodium vivax, ovale and malariae* is much milder and does not cause death, although they cause recurrent malaria which in itself is a debilitating disease.

The malaria parasite is found mostly in tropical and subtropical regions of the world. Breeding in the mosquito is severely hampered in temperatures below 20 °C. Optimal conditions for mosquito breeding are at temperatures around 30 °C together with humidity levels of over 60 per cent. Consequently temperature and humidity largely dictate whether a country is likely to experience year-round malaria, seasonal malaria or localised breakouts.

The severity of malaria and its incidence is governed also by the immunity levels of the host, man. Immunity depends on constant exposure to the malaria-infected mosquito. Hence war and civil disturbances leading to mass migration of refugees, rapid urbanization and development leading to an influx of non-immune workers as well as tourism, all lead to the exposure of non-immune people to the malaria parasite.

Depending on the income of the non-immune person and the time he is due to spend in the malarious area, he can either choose a form of chemical protection which involves the taking of prophylactics, or mechanical protection — an option that is likely to be preferable for the longer term resident.

Since the dawn of history, humans have battled with malaria and although sporadic advances have been made in different fields by the WHO to combat the disease, it now reports a rapidly growing incidence of cases worldwide. This, coupled with the increasing resistance of the parasite to prophylactic and treatment drugs, is putting pressure on the scientific community to develop a vaccine. Although some advances have been made in this field, there is still a long way to go.

The most those of us who are exposed to malaria can do is to arm ourselves with knowledge of what malaria is all about; how to avoid getting it and if you do contract the disease, how to have it treated promptly and correctly.

2. The history of malaria

Historical records show that malaria is an ancient disease which affected early man as well as certain animals.

In contrast with other diseases which have symptoms that have changed over time, the symptoms of malaria have remained the same since they were first recorded more than two thousand years ago.

Malaria in ancient Greece and Rome

The ancient Greeks were well acquainted with malaria from about the year 500 BC when infected slaves may have carried the disease into Greece. To a certain extent, malaria may well have contributed to the breakdown of ancient Greek civilisation.

As early as 46 BC, Hippocrates described the malaria symptoms and differentiated between its various forms. However, he incorrectly assumed that malaria was caused as a result of drinking stagnant water.

Some time later, Columella (c. AD 116) linked it with germs breeding in swampy ground and he believed that malaria was transmitted to man by mosquitoes or gnats.

Malaria did not discriminate when choosing its victims. One famous victim was Alexander the Great. Ancient Rome was seen to be vulnerable to the fever to the extent that *Gei Febris*, the fever goddess, was worshipped for her ability to cure the disease. The fall of Rome has been attributed not only to hedonism and decadence, but also to the debilitating effects of the illness on its citizens.

Three emperors, Hadrian, Vespasian and Titus are believed to have succumbed to malaria, while St Augustine is thought to have contracted it while carrying Christianity's message from Rome to Britain.

Medieval Europe was well acquainted with malaria until land reclamation and improved drainage disrupted the mosquitoes' breeding habits. These habits were further discouraged inadver-

5

tently by the increased building of well-lit and ventilated houses.

Malaria in England

Malaria was commonly known in the English Fens and the marshy Thames Valley. Its more famous English victims included James 1 and Oliver Cromwell. Up until 1859 when the Thames Embankment was built, records show that 5 per cent of admissions to St Thomas' hospital were as a result of malaria.

Theories about malaria

It took a long time for the connection between malaria and swampy ground to be made. Medieval beliefs that planets and comets rained down a fever-poison or that electrical storms were responsible, had to be overcome first.

During the first half of the nineteenth century it was also believed that dew falling on the decks of ships before sunrise would produce small insects that carried the fever. It was further thought that preferred targets were of fair complexion and were fond of alcohol!

From the Middle Ages up until just over 100 years ago, the dominant theory governing malaria transmission concerned the fact that swamp air contained chemical poisons released from rotting wood. To avoid this, houses were built facing away from wetlands and lakes and double-storey houses were preferred as it was thought that the air did not rise much above ground level.

Known in the Middle Ages as "the ague", malaria's connection with marshy ground was entrenched when it was eventually given the latin name that meant "bad air" i.e. *mal'aria*.

Prophylaxis

Malaria prophylaxis at the time involved the use of crudely made mosquito nets and the hanging of garlic and camphor-filled linen bags around the neck.

6

Treatment

Before the discovery of quinine, malaria treatments included lying in steam baths, taking cold dips in the sea, applying blistering equipment, swallowing strychnine, arsenic and large doses of calomel, and the time-honoured application of leeches. Blood-letting was the preferred treatment of fever. Although these were unsuccessful, their use was continued.

The story of quinine

Ever since its acceptance in 1640 as a proven remedy for the disease, the mainstay of malaria treatment to the present day has been quinine. Having observed Peruvians treating malaria successfully, Jesuit priests living in Peru returned to Europe with the bark of a certain tree that when boiled and the water drunk, greatly improved the survival chances of a malaria victim.

Once introduced to Europe, cinchona (as it was then known) became the drug of choice after use by such famous patients as Charles II and the Archduke Leopold.

Despite its bitter taste, and the fact that it sometimes produced deafness, nausea and vomiting, and that its method of action was still mysterious, quinine became known as a miraculous drug.

Its use was linked with serious risks including its association with blackwater fever, an occasional complication of malaria, but known to be one of the commonest causes of death among expatriates in Africa. It is suspected that irregular doses of quinine used as a prophylactic may have caused this much-feared disease.

Today, quinine taken with tetracycline is often the last drug used, after other drugs have failed to quell malaria.

Malaria in the last 100 years

DDT was thought to be the great breakthrough of the past 100 years, not for treatment of malaria, but for its prevention on a mass scale.

Widespread spraying programmes began in the mid-1950s and a marked reduction in the incidence of malaria was experienced in a number of countries. However, it was not until the early 1970s that it was realised to what extent DDT was actually harming the environment.

When it became known that it did not break down into harmless forms but remained harmful for many years and that with ingestion, DDT could be passed along the food chain, the distribution of the chemical was banned in many countries and so the incidence of malaria increased.

The initial decrease of malaria infections in the late 1960s due to DDT went hand in hand with the introduction of mass prophylaxis campaigns, where populations were treated with chloroquine, as in Tanzania. Here an experiment in mass dosage was carried out where the drug was mixed with table salt in an attempt to ensure that everyone was exposed to it.

Again, it took some time before it was realised that chloroquine-resistant strains of the parasite were developing as a result of the sub-curative doses used during such mass drug administration. It was still to be realised that mechanical protection was better than chemical protection, at least on a large scale.

Since the mid-1980s the halting of the disease's spread seems to have become a lost battle. More than 100 million people worldwide are affected by malaria each year and it is regarded as a bigger killer than AIDS.

It is hoped that the development of the new wonder drug derived from the Chinese herb, *qinghao* (artemether), will go a long way towards reducing the fatal effects of malaria.

This, coupled with the eventual arrival of a long-awaited vaccine should reduce the incidence of deaths among the most vulnerable of malaria's victims. Despite these advances, the hope of eradication has now been transmuted to one merely of control by the WHO.

3. The worldwide incidence of malaria

Worldwide, an astounding 270 million new infections develop annually resulting in an estimated one million deaths.

More than 40 per cent of the world's population living in over 100 countries is exposed to the risk of malaria.

Clinical cases are estimated at over 100 million people annually. Over 90 million of these (90 per cent) are in tropical Africa, i.e. south of the Sahara Desert.

Of the overall number of cases reported annually to the WHO from countries excluding Africa, 90 per cent originate from 19 countries only. Some 75 per cent of these are concentrated in nine countries which are listed as follows in decreasing order of incidence:

1) India	4) Sri Lanka	7) Vietnam
2) Brazil	5) Thailand	8) Cambodia
3) Afghanistan	6) Indonesia	9) China

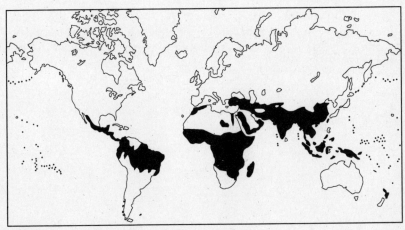

Figure 1: Incidence of malaria in the world

Accurate information on the global incidence of malaria is difficult to obtain because reporting of figures from endemic areas in particular, is incomplete.

At the turn of the century, more than two-thirds of the world's population lived in areas where malaria was endemic. Since 1957, concerted efforts at eradication through chemical means have meant that large parts of the globe are now free from malaria.

However, administrative, political and economic obstacles stand in the way of total eradication. Resistance in the mosquito to insecticide and increasing resistance of the malaria parasite to anti-malarial drugs add enormously to these obstacles. The WHO notes that only a few countries have not as yet reported resistance of *P. falciparum* to the least toxic and most widely-used drug, chloroquine.

Table 1 shows countries in which malaria is reported, its incidence, distribution within the country, type of malaria present and resistance (pages 11–18).

Table 1: Countries in which malaria is reported, its incidence, distribution within the country, type of malaria present and resistance

Country	Time	Altitude	Location	P. vivax	P. falciparum	P. malariae	Resistant to
ASIA							
Afghanistan	May to Nov	Below 2000 m		Predominant	Exists		Chloroquine
Azerbaijan	Not known			Predominant			
Bangladesh	All year		Entire country		Predominant		Chloroquine S/P H/resistant
Bhutan	All year		Ihrir Southern belt	Reported	Predominant		Chloroquine S/P
Burma (see Myanmar)							
Cambodia	All year		Entire country except Phnom Penh		Predominant		Chloroquine, h/resistant S/P
China	July to Nov	Below 1 500 m	North of 33° N	Predominant where falciparum is not	Predominant in Guangxi, Guizhou, Hainan, Yunan and Anhui		Chloroquine
	May to Dec	Below 1 500 m	33° N–25° N				
	All year	Below 1 500 m	South of 25° N				

H/resistant = Highly resistant   S/P = sulphadoxine pyrimethamine

11

Country	Time	Altitude	Location	P. vivax	P. falciparum	P. malariae	Resistant to
Hong Kong	Occasional		Some rural areas				
India	All year		Entire country	Predominant	Exists		Chloroquine H/resistant
Indonesia	All year		Entire country		Predominant		Chloroquine H/resistant S/P resistant
Kampuchea	Present		Present				
Laos	All year		Entire country		Predominant		Chloroquine H/resistant
Malaysia	Not known		Limited areas in deep hinterland		Predominant		Chloroquine H/resistant
Maldives	Not known		Not known		Not known		S/P resistant
Myanmar (Burma)	All year	Below 1 000 m	Entire country		Predominant		Chloroquine H/resistant S/P resistant
Nepal	Not known		Not known				
Pakistan	All year	Below 2 000 m	Entire country		Predominant		Chloroquine
Philippines	All year	Below 600 m	Entire country except urban areas and plains		Predominant		Chloroquine H/resistant
Tajikhistan	Not known			Predominant			

Country	Time	Altitude	Location	P. vivax	P. falciparum	P. malariae	Resistant to
Thailand	All year		Rural, forested, hilly areas only	Predominant			Chloroquine H/resistant;S/P Mefloquine
Vietnam	Not known		Entire country	Predominant	Exists		Chloroquine H/resistant S/P
S. AMERICA							
Argentina	Oct to May	Below 1 200 m	Rural areas	Predominant			
Belize	All year		Belize district urban areas				
Bolivia	All year	Below 2 500 m	Rural areas	Predominant	Some in north-ern areas		Chloroquine S/P
Brazil	All year	Below 900 m	Especially in areas of mining & agriculture		Predominant		Chloroquine H/resistant S/P
Colombia	All year	Below 800 m	Rural areas		Predominant		Chloroquine H/resistant S/P
Costa Rica	All year	Below 800 m	Rural areas	Predominant	Exists		
Dominican Rep	All year		Most parts		Exclusively		
Ecuador	All year	Below 1 500 m	Most parts	Predominant	Exists		Chloroquine
El Salvador	All year		Entire country	Predominant			
French Guiana	All year		Entire country	Not known	Not known		Chloroquine
Guatemala	All year	Below 1 500 m	Entire country	Predominant			Chloroquine
Guyana	All year		Interior	Predominant	Predominant		
Honduras	All year		Entire country	Predominant			Chloroquine

Country	Time	Altitude	Location	P. vivax	P. falciparum	P. malariae	Resistant to
Mexico	All year		Rural areas	Predominant	Mainly in Chiapas		
Nicaragua	June to Dec		Entire country	Predominant			
Panama	All year		Rural and continental areas				Chloroquine
Paraguay	Oct to May		Rural areas	Predominant			
Peru	All year	Below 1 500 m	Entire country	Predominant	Mostly in some parts		Chloroquine S/P
Suriname	All year		Entire country	Exclusively in some parts	Predominant		Chloroquine H/resistant S/P
Venezuela	All year		Rural areas		Predominant		Chloroquine H/resistant
AFRICA							
Algeria	Limited		2 small areas				
Angola	All year		Entire country		Predominant		Chloroquine S/P
Benin	All year		Entire country		Predominant		Chloroquine
Botswana	Nov–May June		Northern parts		Predominant		Chloroquine
Burkina-Faso	All year		Entire country		Predominant		Chloroquine
Burundi	All year		Entire country		Predominant		Chloroquine
Cameroon	All year		Entire country		Predominant		Chloroquine S/P
C. African Rep.	All year		Entire country		Predominant		Chloroquine

Country	Time	Altitude	Location	P. vivax	P. falciparum	P. malariae	Resistant to
Chad	All year		Entire country		Predominant		Chloroquine
Congo	All year		Entire country		Predominant		Chloroquine
Côte D'Ivoire	All year		Entire country		Predominant		Chloroquine
Djibouti	All year		Entire country		Predominant		Chloroquine
Egypt	June to Oct		El Faiyum	Mostly predominant	In El Faiyum area		
			Rural areas of Nile delta Oases and upper Egypt				
Equitorial Guinea	All year		Entire country		Predominant		Chloroquine
Ethiopia	All year	Below 2 000 m	Entire country		Predominant		Chloroquine H/resistant
Gabon	All year		Entire country		Predominant		Chloroquine
Gambia	All year		Entire country		Predominant		Chloroquine
Ghana	All year		Entire country		Predominant		Chloroquine
Guinea	All year		Entire country		Predominant		Chloroquine
Guinea-Bissau	All year		Entire country		Predominant		Chloroquine
Kenya	All year		Entire country		Predominant		Chloroquine H/resistant
Liberia	All year		Entire country		Predominant		Chloroquine H/resistant
Libya	Feb to Aug		Limited risk South West				S/P S/P

15

Country	Time	Altitude	Location	P. vivax	P. falciparum	P. malariae	Resistant to
Malawi	All year		Entire country	Some	Predominant	Some	Chloroquine H/resistant S/P
Mali	All year		Entire country		Predominant		Chloroquine
Mauritania	All year		Entire country except north	Predominant			
Morocco	May to Oct		Rural areas in certain provinces	Exclusively			
Mozambique	All year		Entire country		Predominant		Chloroquine H/resistant S/P
Namibia	Nov to June		Rural north		Predominant		Chloroquine
Niger	All year		Entire country		Predominant		Chloroquine
Nigeria	All year		Entire country		Predominant		Chloroquine
Rwanda	All year		Entire country		Predominant		Chloroquine H/resistant S/P
Senegal	All year		Entire country		Predominant		Chloroquine
Sierra Leone	All year		Entire country		Predominant		Chloroquine
Somalia	All year		Entire country		Predominant		Chloroquine
South Africa	All year	Lower altitudes	N and E Tvl and E Natal		Predominant		Chloroquine
Sudan	All year		Entire country		Predominant		Chloroquine H/resistant

Country	Time	Altitude	Location	P. vivax	P. falciparum	P. malariae	Resistant to
Swaziland	All year		Lowveld areas		Predominant		Chloroquine H/resistant
Tanzania	All year	Below 1 800 m	Entire country		Predominant		Chloroquine H/resistant S/P
Togo	All year		Entire country		Predominant		Chloroquine
Uganda	All year		Entire country		Predominant		Chloroquine
Zaire	All year		Entire country		Predominant		Chloroquine H/resistant
Zambia	Nov to June / All year		Entire country / Zambezi valley		Predominant		Chloroquine H/resistant
Zimbabwe	Nov to June / All year	Below 1 200 m	Zambezi valley		Predominant		Chloroquine
MIDDLE EAST							
Iran	Mar to Nov		Some parts		Predominant		Chloroquine
Iraq	May to Nov	Below 1 500 m	In the north	Predominant	Exists		
Oman	All year		Entire country		Predominant		Chloroquine
Saudi Arabia	All year	Low altitudes	Rural areas		Predominant		Chloroquine
Syria	May to Oct		Entire country	Predominant			
UAE	All year		Foothills and valleys of north	Predominant			
Turkey	Mar to Nov		Many parts	Predominant			
Yemen	All year		Entire country		Predominant		Chloroquine

Country	Time	Altitude	Location	P. vivax	P. falciparum	P. malariae	Resistant to
ISLANDS							
Cape Verde	Limited		Sao Tiago is.				
Comores	All year		Entire country		Predominant		Chloroquine
Haiti	All year	Below 300 m	Suburban and rural areas		Exclusively		
Madagascar	All year		Entire country		Predominant		Chloroquine
Maldives			Disappearing: last 2 cases in 1983				
Mauritius	All year		Rural areas in the north	Exclusively			
Mayotte	All year		Entire island		Predominant		Chloroquine S/P
Papua New Guinea	All year	Below 1 800 m	Entire country		Predominant		Chloroquine
Sao Tome	All year		Entire island		Predominant		Chloroquine
Solomon Is.	All year		All islands		Predominant		Chloroquine
Sri Lanka	All year		Entire country	Predominant	Exists		Chloroquine H/resistant
Vanautu	All year		All islands except Futuna		Predominant		Chloroquine H/resistant S/P

4. The mosquito

More than 3 200 species of mosquito have been identified. Not all carry malaria, but of those which do, some species transmit it to humans more efficiently than others. Only the genus *Anopheles* carries a malaria parasite that can be transmitted to a human being.

Feeding and breeding habits

The adult mosquitoes of both sexes feed on nectar and other fluids, thus it makes good sense to reduce the number of nectar producing plants grown in your environment and to remove residual sources of water where possible. Living or staying near these two sources is likely to produce an excess of mosquitoes if you live in a malarious country.

Mosquitoes always breed in water or damp locations. Eggs are deposited on damp soil or vegetation, in moist tree holes and containers or sometimes directly onto water, from where the larvae hatch.

Optimal breeding temperatures for the mosquito are between 25 °C and 3O °C. They can still breed in temperatures as low as 2O °C but cooler conditions will severely hamper the hatching of larvae. Ideal conditions are in humidity levels greater than 60 per cent.

The majority of mosquitoes hunt and feed at night. Each species has a well-defined activity cycle with some attacking at dusk, others at around midnight and so on.

When do they normally bite?

The female anopheles which carry malaria require a blood-meal in order to feed their developing eggs. They usually bite at night, and often round about dawn and dusk. Despite this preference, it would seem that one can be bitten by mosquitoes in heavily shaded, dark conditions during the day, e.g. dark undergrowth, dark cupboards and corners and places which would perhaps appear to be like night-time conditions.

What kind of activity cycles do they display?

Malaria carrying mosquitoes enter houses at dusk and, after a blood-meal, rest on walls or ceilings, spending one or two days inside before leaving to lay eggs in favourable areas outside. Consequently, the spraying of walls and ceilings would deter this activity. However, mosquito behaviour has been known to become selective so that they avoid walls and ceilings and rest elsewhere.

Their movements and the link with resistance

Mosquitoes are accomplished flyers and can disperse over an area of a few kilometres. However, most kinds remain in rather restricted habitats, usually near to their larval development site. This would explain why when resistance in a person is built up, that resistance is usually only to the type of parasite carried by the mosquitoes living in that area. That same person would not likely be resistant to malaria in a different area.

Reducing your chances of being bitten by changing your environment

It has been suggested that the chance of getting bitten by a malaria-carrying mosquito can be reduced if you ensure that you do not choose holiday accomodation near a large number of children as they usually carry a high proportion of malaria parasites in their bodies when they are infected; neither should you have maize, sisal or bananas or any other dense vegetation growing in your garden or near your house, as these may act as resting sites for mosquitoes.

What does the anopheles mosquito look like?

The anopheles mosquito has dappled wings and, when it is resting, tilts itself head-down at an angle of forty-five degrees. This characteristic stance is in contrast with the horizontal position maintained by most mosquito species.

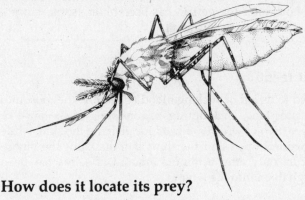

How does it locate its prey?

Anopheles is blind in the dark but seeks its host in response to a combination of chemical and physical stimuli. It has sensors in its two antennae which enable it to detect the stream of carbon dioxide exhaled by its prey.

This allows it to calculate its distance from the prey as it moves towards it through the changing concentrations in the air of warmth, moisture and the ingredients of human sweat.

Human perspiration differs in its content, with that of certain individuals being more desirable to the biting insect than that of others. This may explain to a small extent why certain people get bitten more often than others.

Does the malaria-carrying mosquito make a noise?

In contrast to the relatively high-pitched, loud, characteristic buzz of the mosquito, the malaria-carrying mosquito has a low-pitched almost inaudible hum, unless it is quite close to the ear.

What causes the itchy bite?

A localized sensitivity to saliva from the mosquito causes the itch. The saliva contains an anti-clotting agent which allows the blood-meal to enter the mosquito's stomach without coagulating and becoming indigestible.

The same reaction seems to be present with all types of mosquito but the size of the reaction seems to differ in varying degrees, i.e. some bites may be visible for days after while others disappear about half an hour after the person has been bitten; some cause a lot of itching while others hardly at all.

How does it feed?

Highly adapted to its job of sucking blood efficiently, the mosquito has a proboscis or long, sucking organ, consisting of six hair-like stylets or probes, two of which are used for piercing the skin, while two saw the wound open and the third pair suck out the blood-feed. This occurs only after a minute amount of saliva has been injected through them into the wound.

5. The different types of malaria

The four types of malaria are split into two categories; there are three types which are benign forms: *Plasmodium vivax, malariae* and *ovale* and one malignant form *Plasmodium falciparum*.

The latter parasite is responsible for the majority of deaths caused by malaria, whereas the malaria caused by the first three do not usually cause death, but only debilitating disease, which in some cases can recur over many years.

One reason for the differences in severity can be attributed to the preference of the different parasites for red blood cells at different stages of maturation: *P. vivax* and *P. ovale* invade the younger red blood cells, while *P. malariae* prefers mature blood cells; *P. falciparum* on the other hand is indiscriminate in its choice of red blood cells, hence its form of attack is all-encompassing. This substantially broadens the scope and potential severity of its attack.

The life cycles of the four malarial parasite types are broadly similar, with different stages of development occurring in appropriate female anopheles mosquito hosts as well as in the human host.

The least dangerous form of the disease causes periodic chills and fever but is rarely fatal, hence the term "benign". Despite the term "benign", *vivax* malaria can be fatal in patients who suffer traumatic rupture of the spleen and in those who develop severe anaemia, especially malnourished and debilitated patients.

Old-fashioned terms for the different types of malaria are:

P. vivax	Benign tertian, simple tertian, tertian
P. malariae	Quartan
P. falciparum	Malignant tertian, subtertian, aestivo-autumnal, tropical pernicious.
P. ovale	Ovale tertian

These colloquial names have become largely obsolete.

Plasmodium vivax

After *P. falciparum*, *P. vivax* is the second most widely experienced form of malaria. A serious complication in untreated infections is rupture of the spleen as noted above.

Vivax occurs mostly in the temperate zone as well as in the tropics. It is common in Central America and China where it is responsible for most malaria cases, whereas in West Africa and East Africa it causes only about 2 per cent of malaria cases.

To demonstrate how benign it is, of more than five million cases of a *vivax* malaria epidemic in Sri Lanka in 1969, not one person died.

Moreover, this type of malaria is associated with people of a certain blood type not usually found in Africans.

Characteristically, it causes malaria with frequent relapses if not treated properly, the pattern of which varies in relation to the various strains of *P. vivax*.

The incubation period between the time of the first infected bite to first onset of symptoms is between 12 and 17 days or even up to a year, depending on the strain involved.

The severity of the first attack ranges from mild to severe depending on the immune responses of the host and the degree of parasite infection, i.e. for victims with no immunity, severity is likely to be marked.

Plasmodium ovale

This type of malaria is more commonly encountered in sub-Saharan Africa than the *vivax* type. It has mostly been found in West Africa.

Its symptoms are indistinguishable from those of *vivax* and *malariae*, the other benign types of malaria.

Characteristically, it produces fever spikes every 48–50 hours but this may differ markedly with different cases. If left untreated, or treated inadequately, the infection typically lasts from 18 months to three years although periods of recurrence may be lengthy between attacks.

The severity of the first attack is typically mild with fever attacks lasting from eight to 12 hours.

Incubation from the time of the first infected bite till the onset of symptoms is typically from 16 to 18 days or even longer (depending on the strain involved).

Plasmodium malariae

Also known as *malariae quartain* as its fevers sometimes spike every 72 hours. Its course is not unduly severe but it is notorious for its long persistence in the body if adequate treatment is not given. Its geographical range extends over both tropical and subtropical areas.

The incubation period between the time of the first infected bite and the first onset of symptoms ranges between 18 to 40 days or even longer.

This can present problems in those who for instance get bitten on the last day of their holiday and develop malaria symptoms some five weeks later. Unless one was looking out for malaria, it would be difficult to immediately link the illness with the holiday. This is compounded because the severity of the first attack is usually mild, so it may arouse little suspicion.

The fever cycle usually occurs every 72 hours while the fever lasts for an average of eight to 10 hours.

Malariae does not relapse as happens with *vivax* and *ovale* but rather "recrudesces" or "breaks out" again. With the *malariae* parasite it seems that the infection persists in very low concentrations in the blood. When the concentration increases we say that the infection has "recrudesced". The incidence of break-outs is high and these can last for between three and 50 years.

It is possible for the host to be infected and not develop symptoms for 50 years, as happened in one case where a person who had lived in a malarious area briefly in their youth developed it many years later after spending the rest of their life in non-malarious England.

It is not known what the reason is for such a long, symptom-free period nor has it been confirmed that stress or illness may have a part to play in triggering the disease.

Plasmodium falciparum

Malignant malaria, the killer disease, is caused by the species named *Plasmodium falciparum* which nearly always causes severe, life-threatening malaria in non-immune hosts.

The greater the amount of immunity possessed by the host, the milder the disease is when it does strike. Over 90 per cent of malaria cases and 90 per cent of deaths in Africa are due to *P. falciparum* whereas about 40 per cent of total cases in Asia are due to it.

P. falciparum malaria is the fatal form of malaria which can kill a non-immune person within less than a week or two of a primary attack unless appropriate treatment is given in time.

It takes between six and 14 days for malaria to develop from the time of the first infected bite to the first sign or symptom. In this time the parasite has been multiplying in the liver before being released into the bloodstream and invading the red blood cells.

The typical cycle between fever spikes is usually 48 hours, but with different batches of parasite maturing at different times, these fever spikes are likely to become less obvious and interspersed with other fever spikes, making detection of a pattern difficult.

The severity of the first malaria attack is always the worst in those who have no immunity to malaria. In others with partial immunity the severity of the attack may be less.

Should a relapse occur as a result of inadequate or incorrect treatment of the malaria attack, it will break out again relatively soon, i.e. a few weeks.

6. The symptoms of malaria

The symptoms of malaria are the same today as they were more than two thousand years ago when they were first described. The static nature of malaria symptoms contrasts with other diseases whose symptoms have varied over time.

General symptoms

The symptoms are basically similar for the four types of malaria although the clinical manifestations may differ significantly. In general, the infection is characterised by bouts of fever occurring at regular intervals, alternating with periods of partial recovery with the patient becoming weaker as time goes on.

It is important to note that the classic description is characteristic but *not* universal and variations may be found which typically serve to confuse diagnosis.

In primary attacks, i.e. during the first-ever attack of malaria, bouts of fever may occur daily for the first few days before the fever settles into the characteristic tertian quartan pattern (every 48 or 72 hours).

As bouts continue, the spleen becomes enlarged and tender, and *herpes labialis* (cold sores on the mouth) may appear.

In children the manifestations are often atypical and may be alarming. Paroxysms of fever are not as common as with adults, while headache, nausea, vomiting, abdominal pain, diarrhoea, a sustained fever and convulsions make up a much less characteristic clinical picture.

What can make diagnosis difficult?

Diagnosis is particularly difficult with children who may have high blood levels of parasites but relatively mild symptoms.

Conversely, there may be little or no sign of parasites in the blood and symptoms may be severe.

Misdiagnosis is a serious problem in areas where health workers are not familiar with malaria, or with patients in whom the range of symptoms may not clearly point to malaria.

The three stages of the malaria crisis

The malaria crisis or paroxysm classically comprises a cold stage, a hot stage, and a sweating stage.

1. The cold stage

This can last from 15 minutes to more than an hour. An abrupt onset of chills with distinctive, uncontrollable shivering will develop. There is a feeling of intense cold and the patient shivers from head to foot despite putting on all available clothing and blankets. The teeth may also chatter uncontrollably.

Children may be prone to convulsive fits and vomiting may occur in adults.

If vomiting does happen, remember that dehydration may occur and counter this with extra fluids. Diarrhoea may also be an accompanying symptom.

Note whether any medicines taken have had time to be absorbed — a good rule of thumb should be about 30 minutes on an empty stomach or up to 45 minutes on a stomach with some food in it. However, medical opinion is divided on this subject.

2. The hot stage

Shivering is followed by the "hot stage" which lasts for between two and six hours, during which the patient suffers a sensation of great heat. Clothes are discarded and the pulse becomes strong and bounding. There is high fever (40–41 °C), intense headache, malaise and often abdominal pain, vomiting, thirst and frequent urination as well as muscle, joint and back pains.

3. The sweating stage

This stage usually lasts for between one to four hours during which the patient may sweat profusely, saturating clothes and bedding. He or she often falls into a deep sleep and awakes exhausted but otherwise quite well. The temperature falls back to normal and the symptoms disappear.

Strength returns slowly until the next attack. Should the malaria continue over a number of days, a cyclic pattern will emerge with symptoms occurring on every third day or so. However, most people obtain treatment before this cyclic pattern has a chance to emerge.

In some malaria infections, the fever can be more or less continuous without the cyclic paroxysms. Symptoms may be minimal or absent in persons who have developed a strong immunity against malaria. They may exhibit only fever.

Symptoms of *Plasmodium falciparum*

The incubation period of *P. falciparum* malaria is usually between seven to 12 days and is seldom over 28 days (although cases of longer duration have been recorded).

The onset of malaria may be distinctive and unmistakeable in some persons while in others it may be slow and non-specific, causing medical care not to be sought for several days. However, the first attack of *falciparum* in non-immune patients is the most serious and dangerous as the host has no immunity against the disease and is at his or her most vulnerable. These patients may have a "flu-like" illness, with fever, headache, dizziness, malaise, aches and pains, but shaking chills and high fever are not always present.

Jaundice, which is not uncommon, may be mistaken for viral hepatitis. Associated symptoms vary, but may include nausea, vomiting and a bronchitic cough. Diarrhoea is not uncommon.

The character of the fever, its symptoms and course are irregular and variable. At first, fever is intermittent and irregular; later it is characterised by numerous peaks representing the activity of different groups of parasites. The rigor (sudden chill with shivering before fever) is definitely a danger signal, indicating the need for immediate treatment.

Anaemia arises from the destruction of the red blood cells by the malaria parasite. The *falciparum* parasite shows no discrimination in blood cells and will destroy cells of any age as opposed to the *vivax* parasite which destroys only young or immature blood cells.

This blanket approach explains why the patient will deteriorate far more quickly than he would with the other forms of malaria. The destruction of the red blood cells causes them to stick together, forming small clots which block capillaries, leading to areas of defective oxygenation in many tissues. It is also thought that a toxic substance is produced by *falciparum* that may possibly adversely affect the metabolism of the tissue cells.

Taken together, the results of a *falciparum* infection can be sudden, grave and can develop without warning. These complications include cerebral malaria. (see section on Complications, page 49)

The recurring malarias

Vivax and *ovale* types of malaria recur because the parasite incubates in the liver for long periods after infection and then appears in the blood, causing renewed symptoms on relapse. This may explain why the patient can undergo attacks long after he has left the malarious area.

Symptoms of *Plasmodium vivax*

The variable incubation lasts between nine to 15 days after which a classic three-stage attack cycle begins.

Vivax is characterised by a primary attack followed by relapses until the patient is cured. It is a serious illness that can lead to anaemia and debility but it is not life-threatening.

In the primary attack, parasites mature on alternate days, causing a fever roughly every 24 hours, each time they mature.

In secondary or relapse attacks, the parasites mature on the same day causing fever at 48 hour intervals. By the second week, the spleen has enlarged and is often tender. The spleen may rupture as a result, but this is said to be rare.

Anaemia results from the destruction of the red blood cells and this may be severe in children. In severe cases, jaundice may develop. It has not been proven that this effect will be compounded when the patient may have had hepatitis or any other form of liver dysfunction.

Relapses usually fall into two categories: early, eight to 10 weeks after the attack and late, between 30 to 40 weeks after the attack. It is unusual to see relapses more than three years after the infection. The reason for this phenomenon is not known.

Symptoms of *Plasmodium malariae* (quartan)

Incubation is between 15 and 40 days and is followed by a three stage cycle of similar severity to that in *vivax* infection but which occurs at 72 hour intervals. Patients have been known to experience relapses up to 20 years after the primary infection.

This infection can be completely wiped out by adequate retreatment so that relapses do not occur. It is not life-threatening although it can cause kidney complications.

Symptoms of *Plasmodium ovale* (tertian)

This is much milder than a *vivax* infection, and it exhibits similar symptoms. In the primary attack, the fever occurs at 48 hour intervals.

7. The life cycle of the malaria parasite

After a mosquito carrying malaria parasites has bitten a person, the parasites have been shown to disappear from the outer (peripheral) blood supply within half an hour, only to return to it six to 16 days later. During this week-long latent period the malarial patient cannot re-infect a "clean" mosquito if he or she is bitten again.

Soon after entering the human bloodstream, the parasites "hide" in the host's liver, where they are largely immune to drug therapy. At this point, a drug such as Proguanil (Paludrine) may be effective in preventing further development of the parasite.

After lodging in the liver for six to 16 days, the parasites multiply and are released into the bloodstream. There they invade red blood cells where they multiply and are released again into the bloodstream where the process continues.

As it continues, the infection leads to a progressive increase of parasites in the blood (parasitaemia) until the process is slowed down by the immune response of the host, is blocked by appropriate treatment, or ultimately overwhelms the system and results in death.

This development cycle takes 48 hours in tertian malaria (i.e. in three different types of parasite — *falciparum, vivax and ovale*) to 72 hours in quartan malaria (*malariae*).

P. vivax, P. malariae and *P. ovale* are very specific in terms of the red blood cells they attack. This is one of the reasons why they result in correspondingly less severe pathological changes and manifestations than happens with *P. falciparum*.

P. falciparum invades any red blood cell resulting in severe and sudden symptoms in some individuals.

Infections of *P. vivax* and *P. ovale* may remain in a dormant phase on entering the liver and only begin active division after a genetically predetermined interval, causing the characteristic relapses of these infections.

The mosquito bites its victim.

Malaria parasite "eggs" (sporozoites) in the salivary gland
are injected into the person's bloodstream.

The parasite heads for the liver cells where it
stays in an incubatory phase for between six and 15 days.
P. ovale and *P. vivax* stay dormant in the liver for much longer.

In the liver form the parasite develops into another form (schizonts)
which, in turn, mature and release a differentiated form of parasite
(merozoite) into the bloodstream where they invade red blood cells.
At this point the merozoites reinfect liver cells causing relapses
(not with *P. falciparum*).

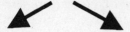

Some of the newly released
merozoites are differentiated
into gametocytes.

In the bloodstream (the bloodstream
form) they mature into schizonts and
are released as merozoites from the
red blood cell when it ruptures. This
causes fever.

These, while circulating in the
bloodstream are ingested when
a mosquito takes a blood-feed
from the person.

The released merozoites invade
new blood cells, causing the fever.
The process continues until death
or appropriate medication kills the
parasite.

A further form of parasite development and differentiation
takes place inside the mosquito resulting in the beginning
of the cycle again when the parasite lodges in the salivary
glands of the mosquito and gets injected into humans
when they are bitten again.

N.B. Different drugs are effective at different stages in the parasite's life cycle.

Figure 2: The life cycle of the malaria parasite

As the parasites continue to multiply, they rupture red blood cells releasing more parasites. In established infections, this usually happens at once resulting in the sudden onset of fever.

When a certain amount of blood cells are destroyed, anaemia with jaundice may develop.

Characteristically, the spleen and liver may become enlarged as a result of increased debris from the digested and ruptured red blood cells.

8. What to do if malaria is suspected

Malaria is unique in its propensity to pass rapidly from a mild illness whose treatment is relatively simple, to a catastrophic state in which the outlook is virtually hopeless.

Failure to consider malaria in diagnosis, or the inability to recognise parasites in a blood smear can prove fatal.

Symptoms

The signs that should alert you to a possibility of malaria include those that are described under the section on symptoms (page 27).

However, remember that in some cases, fever may not be present, while only diarrhoea and/or vomiting may be present. If you feel unwell, especially "fluey", and you have recently been, or are living in, a country where malaria is endemic, you should first of all consider the possibility of malaria.

Testing

Rather test for it and come up with negative results than assume that something else is wrong with you. However, to complicate matters, also remember that if you are taking prophylactics, your test is likely to come up negative anyway.

Time is of the essence

Remember that time is of the essence. If malaria is suspected early in the evening, and it is decided that a doctor will be consulted only the next morning, a whole 12 hours will have elapsed during which time the parasite can multiply and significantly weaken someone who is at risk, i.e. a baby or small child, a pregnant woman, or a non-immune person.

What if you cannot get hold of a doctor?

It is best to consult whatever medical facilities are likely to be open at the time or to take the decision to treat for malaria yourself. If you take that decision you need to have on hand one of the treatment drugs recommended for that particular region.

It is essential that you seek medical advice as soon as possible to confirm the diagnosis and to confirm that you are taking the correct drug regimen. If medical help is not available, your best course would be to take the entire course of treatment as prescribed in the package insert of the drug.

If your condition worsens then you can assume one of two things: you are suffering from malaria but the drug you have taken has not worked and you should take a more powerful drug. Or, you are not suffering from malaria at all, but rather from some other disease on which the drugs you have taken have no effect.

What drugs should you have on hand?

The first line of attack in a malarial country would usually be chloroquine although in many countries it has lost its effectiveness due to the development of resistance. Refer to page 90 for the first line drug of choice for treatment.

Fever is likely to persist for as long as 48–72 hours before an improvement is likely to be noticeable. With Fansidar it has been observed that a second fever spike on the second or third day after commencing medication often occurs. This may lead one to think that the medication has not worked.

Between the time the dose was given and the next morning there may still be some effect of a failed or inadequate drug, enough to hold off multiplication of the parasite until a doctor is consulted.

The doctor would have to advise you whether to continue with the drug, how to watch out for signs that the drug was not working and when to come back for a further blood test to ascertain that the parasite had been eradicated from the bloodstream.

Other measures to take to help minimise the effects of malaria

Other measures that should be taken include giving anti-fever drugs, sponging with tepid water (not cold or hot), and removal of clothes during the hot stage. It would also be useful to monitor symptoms over time.

If vomiting is present note when the drug was given and whether enough time elapsed (one hour) before the vomiting occurred.

Drug administration and absorption

Medical opinion is divided on the specific time that should be allowed to elapse after the medicine has been taken, and before vomiting occurs, to judge if absorption has taken place. Absorption depends on whether food was present in the stomach at the time of ingestion or not; on the metabolic rate of the particular patient and on the drug that is administered.

If insufficient time for absorption occurred, then the dose must be re-administered. Overdosage has different effects with different drugs. If vomiting is already established or if the patient is prone to vomiting, give the patient an anti-nausea, anti-vomiting drug about 45 minutes before you are due to give the medication.

Unfortunately no treatment drugs are available in suppository form at present — something which would go a long way to overcoming the problem of vomiting and having to put the patient on a drip.

Remember that if diarrhoea is present as well, to rehydrate the patient adequately.

Table 2: Rehydration therapy

Large amounts of fluid or oral rehydrate solution (ORS) are to be taken in cases of diarrhoea to ensure adequate rehydration ecommended by the WHO)

Children less than two years:
  1/4 to 1/2 cup (50-100 ml) after each loose stool
Children two to 10 years:
  1/2 to 1 cup (100 ml to 200 ml)after each loose stool
Older children to adults:
  Unlimited amounts

If ORS is not available, make up a home-made solution:
  Six level tablespoons of sugar
  One level teaspoon of salt
  Dissolve the above in one litre of clean, boiled water.
Drink this in amounts as indicated above for ORS.

9. Diagnosis

Most deaths in short stay travellers which are due to malaria are likely to occur after their return to their country of origin. The single biggest contributory factor in the death of such a person is *the lack of prompt and accurate diagnosis.*

Indeed, in 1993 the family of a man who died of malaria in an English hospital after returning from Kenya, successfully sued the hospital for failure to diagnose malaria. The award granted was £900,000.

Doctors in non-endemic areas may not be alert to a diagnosis of malaria, nor be familiar with the disease. Even if blood smears are taken for some other reason, malarial parasites may not be recognised by lab technicians as they will not be looking for them, nor will they have any experience in recognising them.

Guard against the possibility of your blood test being sent away to another hospital for analysis. Inquire how long it will be before you have results. One hapless person returning to the UK who suspected he might have malaria, had the foresight to have his blood tested. Unfortunately, he received his results three days later, during which time he may easily have died, had his results been positive.

This applies in particular to school children who return to school in England or some other European country after spending a holiday with their parents in a malaria endemic area. School masters and school doctors need to be very alert in their diagnosis of fevers in such children on their return to school.

One wise rule is to make sure the returning traveller is equipped with an effective treatment drug in case they meet with any difficulty or delay in obtaining the drug in their home country.

Be on your guard if you or your visitors leave the country and within a month to six weeks come down with what seems like flu. It is so easy to forget that you have been in an endemic area and that malaria might be the cause of your illness.

Basing diagnosis on a blood smear

If there is any hint of suspicion on the doctor's part that malaria may be present, he should begin anti-malarial therapy, *even if parasites are not found in the blood smear*. It has been known for doctors who are not familiar with malaria to refuse to treat for malaria despite all the classic symptoms being present, unless they can see parasites in the blood smear.

It may be that the parasites at an early stage of development in the body may not be visible in the peripheral bloodstream, making a blood smear inconclusive. If this is the case, examinations of blood smears taken at frequent intervals may be necessary to establish a diagnosis.

It is not easy to say exactly, but two to three blood smears taken every 8–12 hours should be sufficient to confirm a diagnosis.

To further complicate the issue, a positive blood smear taken from a feverish patient living in an endemic region does not conclusively implicate malaria as the cause of the illness. This is because the patient may show no symptoms but may have parasites circulating in the blood anyway. His immunity may be such that the infection is under control and not causing disease. In such a case, the patient's fever may be due to other infectious agents.

In addition, patients with cerebral malaria may display scanty parasite counts while many children with high parasite counts may display fairly mild symptoms.

Patients who have been taking prophylactics need to tell their doctor this, as these will very likely mask the presence of parasites in the blood and result in a seemingly negative blood smear.

The conclusion therefore is that a negative blood smear does not exclude malaria and a positive blood smear does not necessarily confirm a diagnosis of malaria.

A good rule of thumb to apply is the following: Malaria should be suspected by medical personnel in anyone with a fever who has recently been in a malaria endemic area.

The doctor should admit the patient to hospital for drug administration by drip if the patient is unable to keep down medication given by mouth.

Admission to the intensive care unit should be made if the patient has difficulty in talking, sitting up, standing or walking without any other obvious cause such as unexplained heavy bleeding, the passage of small quantities of, or no urine, or the passage of dark urine; a change of behaviour, confusion or drowsiness; altered consciousness or coma; jaundice and/or severe anaemia; circulatory collapse or shock; difficulty in breathing.

Severe *falciparum* malaria is a medical emergency demanding the highest level of care and treatment available, preferably in an intensive care unit.

What you should tell your doctor

You should tell him or her whether you have been travelling in or visiting a malarial area and when you were there. Your doctor also needs to know whether you have had any symptoms in the past that may have been attributable to malaria and whether you have any history of liver disorder, as this may complicate matters tremendously.

Inform your doctor whether you are likely to be pregnant and whether you are breastfeeding. Tell him or her which prophylactic drugs, if any, you had been taking for malaria and for how long, and whether you took the full dosage conscientiously. Also say whether you have attempted any treatment of your condition.

If your doctor is unfamiliar with malaria, ask him or her to make contact with the Tropical Diseases Institute in the country you are in for further advice.

Diagnostic criteria guideline

These are the criteria your doctor is likely to use in assessing which drug should be used in treating you for malaria.

a) Microscopic confirmation.　　　[ ] positive　[ ] negative
b) Presence of fever.　　　　　　[ ] yes　　　[ ] no
c) Additional signs and symptoms (eliminate other diseases that may cause high fever)
　　　　　　　　　　　　　　　[ ] diarrhoea
　　　　　　　　　　　　　　　[ ] vomiting
　　　　　　　　　　　　　　　[ ] anaemia
　　　　　　　　　　　　　　　[ ] other (name them)
d) Is there chloroquine resistance in the place where the patient is likely to have been bitten?

If yes, treat with:
- Sulfadoxine-pyrimethamine (Fansidar) (if patient is not allergic to sulfa) unless there is also resistance in that area to sulfadoxine pyrimethamine.
- Halofantrine (Halfan), but not if the patient is pregnant or breastfeeding
- Mefloquine (Lariam), but not if the patient is pregnant or desires to fall pregnant in the next three months
- Quinine and tetracycline if malaria is severe (no tetracycline if patient is pregnant or younger than eight) or if the patient has come from an area with sulfadoxine-pyrimethamine and mefloquine resistance. If no, treat with chloroquine.

  (Use of chloroquine as a first line drug still appears justified under current circumstances in the setting where resistance is still low.)

NB. It is important to note that each case is individual. Factors such as past illness, present condition, known resistance of the parasite, availability of other drugs and level of medical care, all need to be weighed and considered. Bearing this in mind, this section should only be used as a guideline as to what the doctor might consider when weighing a particular case.

Follow-up

Following therapy and within 48 hours, there should be a marked decrease in parasite count on the blood smear, coupled with reduction in temperature and other signs and symptoms e.g. vomiting and diarrhoea.

Children under five in an endemic area

If in a child under five there has been in the past two or three days:

- ✧ a history of fever
- ✧ a temperature of 37,5 °C or more
- ✧ the child has been in an endemic area

then regard the illness as malaria and treat accordingly.

If there is another simultaneous diagnosis, eg. tonsillitis, that must be treated as well.

More sophisticated care is required if there are

✧ neurological manifestations, i.e. altered or decreased state of consciousness, coma, delirium, confusion, dulling of sensations, convulsions
✧ persistent vomiting
✧ persistent diarrhoea
✧ temperature 39 °C or higher with dry skin and other signs of dehydration
✧ hypothermia (35,7 °C or lower)
✧ severe anaemia
✧ jaundice
✧ pregnancy with fever
✧ failure to respond to treatment within two days
✧ reactions to drugs interfering with normal daily routine.

Treatment failure

Treatment with a particular drug may fail because the parasites from that particular region may be resistant to the drug. There are strong possibilities that failure may occur with chloroquine and sulfadoxine-pyrimethamine (Fansidar), and much smaller chances of failure may exist where halofantrine (Halfan) and mefloquine (Lariam) are used for the same reason.

It is usual to use another drug for treatment rather than the drug which has previously been taken in prophylactic form. In other words, if chloroquine has been used as a prophylactic and been taken conscientiously, and malaria still persists, it more than likely means that that particular parasite is resistant to the drug.

In addition, inadequate or insufficient earlier treatment may have caused selection of parasites in the patient's body. Say for instance he had malaria and was treated with halofantrine (Halfan), but took insufficient dosage, the malaria would be controlled temporarily but in a suppressed form.

When it re-emerges, the parasites then active are more likely to be those that survived the first treatment by halofantrine (Halfan). Consequently, another drug should be given.

10. Testing for malaria

What should the test show the doctor?

A test that is positive for malaria will show the presence of *Plasmodium* parasites in blood smears. Thick smears will reveal the presence of parasites, while thin smears will reveal which of the four types of plasmodium is attacking the patient. However, the thin smear test is not as sensitive as the thick smear test and may miss low-grade infections.

In a non-immune person a smear will indicate an adequate estimate of the number of circulating parasites and the intensity of the infection. A "plus one" (+1) infection indicates low severity, (++) plus two and (+++) plus three indicate increasing severity while (++++) plus four indicates that the patient should be in intensive care.

In a person with some immunity, there is no absolute relationship between the number of parasites observed and the severity of the infection, as the person may already be harbouring parasites in his blood without being symptomatic.

However, if *falciparum* infection is suspected, treatment should proceed without waiting for confirmation.

A dangerous infection may be present in patients with a negative blood test, especially when they have taken inadequate prophylactic antimalarial drugs or have been treated with some antibacterial agents or with antimalarials. This is because the drugs tend to mask the presence of the parasite in the blood, although the parasite infestation may still be low.

It is still a mystery among doctors that patients with heavy parasite infestation can show few symptoms while those with low or undetectable parasites can manifest typical symptoms. Hence, although the test is very useful, it should not be relied upon absolutely when symptoms are otherwise indicative of malaria.

The best time to have a test

For practical purposes, as soon as possible, but even better if it is during a fever spike.

Does the hospital do the test?

Inquire when you can expect to receive the results of the blood tests. For instance in the United Kingdom, not all hospitals are equipped to test malaria and may have to send the sample away to a laboratory which analyses it. In such cases it has been known that the results were returned to the patient some three days later. If the patient did have malaria he may well have been dead by then.

Types of test

Useful laboratory tests that the patient can ask the doctor for, include malaria parasite, platelet and white cell counts as well as measurements of haematocrit or haemoglobin, serum electrolytes and urea or creatinine.

How is the test taken?

The technician should prick the patient's finger with a sterile lancet (see that the packet is opened in front of you) and for a thick blood smear, allow a drop of blood to fall on a clean glass slide which should then be allowed to dry before being stained and then examined under the microscope.

Depending on which country you are in and on facilities available, tests can take between 15 minutes to an hour before results are known. Every effort should be made to obtain test results as soon as possible as delay can prove fatal, especially if many hours have elapsed since the onset of malaria.

Taking your own smear

If you are in a situation where you need to take a smear at a particular time because you suspect you are at the height of the infection, or because doctor's laboratories are closed, you could take your own slide by pricking your finger with a sterile lancet or needle, after first cleaning your finger with a surgical spirit swab (or methylated spirits) and letting it dry. You will need to have clean, sterile glass slides (obtainable from medical equipment companies). Allow the slide to dry.

What to do when test results are negative and you still suspect you have malaria

The general rule is to go ahead and treat for malaria if in any doubt at all. Once treatment is administered, parasites that are still in the blood will take two to three days to disappear so there is no point in testing after treatment.

However, if after 48 hours symptoms are still being displayed, there is a strong chance that the treatment has not worked. At this point it is wise to test again.

After adequate treatment, the patient should be tested one week or so afterwards to confirm that parasites are not visible in the blood.

It must be noted that there is a difference between an infected person and a diseased person, as far as malaria is concerned. A person may be infected with the parasite and have it detectable in his blood, but due to immunity, may not display any symptoms. On the other hand, a person may be infected and become diseased as a result of inadequate immunity. Hence those who are infected without being diseased are important links in the passing on of the disease.

11. Treatment

The most important aspects of treatment

✧ prompt and effective treatment with antimalarials
✧ correction of fluid and electrolyte levels if there has been a fluid loss
✧ correction of hypoglycaemia or low blood sugar, especially in diabetics and pregnant women
✧ correction of anaemia
✧ treatment of concurrent infection if one exists

Bear in mind that statistics show that nearly all deaths in short term travellers afflicted by malaria are caused by the lack of prompt and accurate medical care.

When to treat for malaria

If *P. falciparum* is suspected, even if test results are not yet available or are negative, if the patient has fever or any of the other signs of malaria (see page 27), antimalarial treatment must be given. If another illness is suspected at the same time, treat for that as well.

The most important aim in treatment is to bring the level of parasites present in the blood under control as quickly as possible by the administration of rapidly acting drugs. This presents little difficulty except in *P. falciparum* malaria where the progression of the disease is extremely rapid.

Because of the complicated nature of the drug treatment, the subject will be covered in an appendix. It is intended that in all cases where medical help is available the patient should attempt to obtain it and not treat himself.

However, situations may arise where medical help is not available and a limited amount of information regarding the right and wrong drugs to take, is likely to be better than no information at all.

Similarly, even where medical care is available, conflicting advice offered to the patient may cause him to wish to read his own information regarding drug treatment without having to seek out vast medical tomes in doing his own research. This is where the information presented in the appendix is intended to assist the reader.

Information in the appendix covers the different types of drugs available for malaria treatment; side effects and contra-indications. Suggestions are also made regarding complications such as how to treat fever, diarrhoea and vomiting.

12. The complications of malaria

There are two directions malaria can take. One is uncomplicated malaria where aching joints, fever, headache and possibly nausea characterise the disease. All that needs to happen in this case is for the disease to be cured in time, either through medication or through the individual's own immune response if he has some immunity.

However, it is also possible for complications to occur. Those listed below are all potentially serious and must be treated quickly and efficiently otherwise they may tip the balance towards death. It is important that the doctor treating the patient recognises these complications as part of malaria and treats them accordingly.

Vomiting

This is a complication in the sense that it makes it impossible for necessary medication to be absorbed. Coupled with high fever, repeated vomiting also leads to dehydration (see page 38). This complication develops especially rapidly in small children.

Diarrhoea

This is characterised by the frequent passing of stools containing blood, mucous and blood cells. Again, if not controlled, this condition can lead to potentially fatal dehydration, especially if compounded by the presence of vomiting.

Choleraic malaria

A condition in which profuse watery diarrhoea, nausea and vomiting occur. There are muscular cramps and the diarrhoea may be progressive. Dehydration is of major concern.

Dehydration

Acute fever, vomiting, diarrhoea and anorexia all make dehydration worse. Adequate rehydration and the assurance of fluid intake are important determinants of clinical recovery, especially in young children. Failure to rehydrate may result in shock and kidney failure.

Jaundice

This is a condition which must be monitored, as it arises from the destruction of red blood cells by the malaria parasites. The remains of the destroyed blood cells collect in the blood faster than they can be removed by the body's cleansing organs — the liver and the spleen.

One of the excess waste products is bilirubin which stains the whites of the eyes and the skin (especially the palms of the hands) yellow, and is passed out in the urine giving it a brownish colour, sometimes even turning it black.

The best way to treat this kind of jaundice is to treat the malaria.

Enlargement of the spleen

Like the liver, the spleen acts as a blood filter and when malaria strikes it works overtime to clear the destroyed blood cells in the blood. Repeated exposure to malaria and thus a regular and heavy workload for the spleen results in enlargement and hardening which is especially palpable in young children.

The fact that it is enlarged is not bad in itself and it usually subsides after effective treatment. The enlargement is thought not to affect the future workings of the spleen.

Acute kidney failure

Acute kidney failure may occur with *P. falciparum* malaria. The clinical features include confusion, restlessness, incoherence, jaundice and fever as well as decreased urine output.

It can be counteracted with adequate malaria treatment. The patient may need to be put on a dialysis machine. It is difficult to predict which cases of *P. falciparum* malaria will result in acute kidney failure.

Adverse drug interactions

If you have been treated unsuccessfully and you then go to a different doctor for more treatment, toxic reactions may arise from adverse drug interactions possibly leading to further delay in appropriate treatment and on the whole complicating the possibility of a positive outcome.

Acute respiratory distress syndrome (pulmonary oedema)

This may be caused by careless intravenous re-hydration during severe *falciparum* infection. However, it may also arise before intravenous therapy has commenced. In many cases the patient needs to be put on a respirator until it improves.

Cerebral malaria

Cerebral malaria must be seen as an emergency, as once a coma sets in, deterioration is very rapid and the patient may die before intravenous drips can be set up (see section on cerebral malaria page 68).

Blackwater fever

This formerly common and extremely dangerous complication involves the presence of blood in the urine, hence its name. It is associated with endemic *falciparum* malaria and is most often found in non-immune residents of malarious areas who have had a history of repeated clinical attacks which have been inadequately treated or suppressed by quinine. Cases can range from mild to severe with recovery quite possible in the milder cases.

The person who is more likely to suffer from blackwater fever tends to be in a state of hypersensitivity brought on by the presence of incompletely suppressed *falciparum* malaria. The syndrome may be triggered by a chill, exhaustion or injury.

It is an illness that is rarely seen these days. The literature seems to point to a link between inadequate administration of quinine as a prophylactic in the days before synthetic antimalarials were available. This would seemingly explain why there was a much greater incidence of blackwater fever in days gone by.

Convulsions

If a child is prone to convulsions, and malaria is suspected, the doctor must be informed.

On the other hand if the child is not prone to convulsions, it should still be borne in mind that convulsions can occur especially in high levels of fever. They are also a feature of cerebral malaria.

Anaemia

Anaemia is an inevitable result of malaria and its severity is proportional to the intensity of infection.

In some areas, many patients, particularly children, are already anaemic from other causes or from repeated previous attacks of malaria even before they develop severe malaria. This may be alleviated by blood transfusion, although in areas where blood is not routinely screened for HIV, this procedure can be risky.

A known blood donor should rather be sought if possible and appropriate measures should be taken to avoid over-transfusion.

Severe anaemia is a life-threatening complication. Treatment comprises rapid and effective clearance of parasites and transfusion when necessary. A particular trap is that these children may appear quite well, but if chloroquine is used in a region with possible chloroquine resistance, it is essential that the child's progress be followed closely to ensure complete clearance, for drug failure may lead to a rapid and disastrous deterioration. (See also anaemia in pregnancy, page 56.)

Hypoglycaemia

Hypoglycaemia can be a complication in patients who are given quinine or quinidine intravenously or intramuscularly. It is most grave in pregnant women, a group which seems to be prone to low blood sugar.

Another high risk group is young children with severe malaria disease.

As hypoglycaemia may be confused with other symptoms and signs of severe malaria, blood glucose must frequently be checked, especially in the high-risk groups. It is also a frequent complication in African children.

Hypoglycaemia requires immediate specific treatment to prevent permanent brain damage. It causes confusion, coma and convulsions which closely resemble cerebral malaria. Treatment is intravenous using a concentrated sugar solution until the patient can take fluid and foods by mouth.

Blood glucose must be measured on admission and regularly thereafter in any child with any feature of severe malaria and in all pregnant women with malaria. In the absence of a means of testing blood sugar, hypoglycaemia should be assumed in any comatose child with malaria and treated appropriately.

Shock

This condition is characterised by vascular collapse and extreme coldness of the surface of the body. The temperature is subnormal and blood pressure is low. If untreated the condition is fatal.

13. Malaria in pregnancy

Pregnant women should avoid going into malarious areas if at all possible. If this is unavoidable, they should diligently guard against being bitten by mosquitoes and seek medical help immediately they suspect any illness.

Complications in pregnancy such as miscarriage and stillbirth as well as death of the newborn are greatly enhanced by the infection of the mother and contribute to high maternal death rates in tropical malarious areas.

It is extremely important that medical help should be sought immediately malaria is suspected and treatment with an effective antimalarial must always be given.

Avoiding mosquito bites is always prudent, pregnant or not. Use of bednets, mosquito coils and window screens, the elimination of domestic breeding sites and going indoors after dusk can considerably lessen exposure.

Table 3: Advice to be given by prescribers to pregnant women and women of childbearing potential

Pregnant women	
1.	Malaria in a pregnant woman increases the risk of maternal death, neonatal death, miscarriage and stillbirth.
2.	Do not go to a malarious area unless absolutely necessary.
3.	Be extra diligent in the use of measures to protect against mosquito bites.
4.	Take chloroquine and proguanil (Paludrine) prophylaxis.
5.	Do not take mefloquine (Lariam) or doxycycline (Vibramycin) prophylaxis.
6.	Seek medical help immediately if malaria is suspected, and take emergency standby treatment (quinine is the drug of choice) only if no medical help is immediately available. Medical help must still be sought as soon as possible after standby treatment.

What are the risks of getting malaria in pregnancy?

Pregnant women are more likely to contract malaria infections than women who are not pregnant despite the fact that they may be resistant to the malaria parasite. Moreover, if and when they do become infected, they will display a higher parasite count in their blood.

Lowered resistance or increased vulnerability

Pregnancy reduces a mother's resistance to malaria, especially in early pregnancy. This vulnerability slowly reduces after the 24th week.

Of course, the non-immune mother who is, for instance, newly arrived in an endemic area, will be as vulnerable as any other non-resistant person. However, pregnancy will complicate malaria and its treatment, should she contract it. This is why women who are pregnant or who are planning to become pregnant, are advised not to visit endemic countries.

In some circumstances, *P. falciparum* infection may be more severe during pregnancy, presumably as a result of depressed maternal immunity.

The risk of severe or fatal disease is greatest for the presumably resistant mother in areas of unstable transmission, where malaria is not transmitted all year round but only when conditions are favourable, such as during the rains or periods of hotter temperature.

In contrast, pregnant women in areas of Africa with highly endemic malaria are generally not at greater risk of severe disease, but their susceptibility to malaria does increase during pregnancy, particularly among women who are pregnant for the first time and who suffer from anaemia and the various complications of chronic parasite infection.

Risks during a first pregnancy

A woman pregnant for the first time is more likely to develop malaria than she will in later pregnancies. If a woman does develop malaria during her first pregnancy, she seems to develop some protection against malaria in her later pregnancies.

Malaria is particularly damaging to pregnant women during their first and second gestations when it can damage the fetus.

A woman in her first pregnancy should therefore be especially alert for malarial symptoms and signs of possible complications and seek treatment promptly.

What are the side effects of getting malaria in pregnancy?

Falciparum malaria during pregnancy poses a threat to the life of the mother and the fetus and may lead to severe anaemia and fetal growth retardation.

The impact of malaria during pregnancy on later development during infancy and childhood is not known.

Anaemia caused by malaria in pregnancy

Anaemia in pregnancy can cause fetal death, intrauterine growth retardation, low birth weight and premature delivery. Women who are pregnant for the first time and in their third trimester are at particular risk of severe anaemia and sometimes even death.

Anaemia among mothers who contract malaria is most common between the 16th and 24th weeks and occurs when malaria parasites destroy red blood cells. Treatment of malaria in early pregnancy, when the mother's resistance is lowest, can prevent development of anaemia later in pregnancy.

Giving iron or folic acid is of little benefit to the mother if malaria parasites continue to destroy red blood cells.

Severe anaemia is aggravated by loss of blood during delivery.

Transplacental infection of the fetus

Premature or false labour is common in mothers infected with malaria. It is possible for the malaria parasite to infect the fetus via the placenta, resulting in its being born with malaria.

Transplacental infection of the fetus is far more common in non-immune mothers than in indigenous populations in malarious areas. A relationship exists between low birth weight and malarial infection of the placenta.

Although it may sound rather innocuous, low birth weight is an unnecessary handicap for an infant who may have to fight against other handicaps at birth such as jaundice or breathing problems. Depending on circumstances and neonatal equipment available, the infant's chance of survival may be severely threatened.

Triggering a latent infection

The stress of childbirth may awaken a latent malaria infection in the semi-immune mother. Although her body may have kept the infection under control during pregnancy, the birth process may trigger the infection to the point where her body can no longer fight it and full-blown malaria develops. Either rapid treatment of acute infection or effective prophylaxis is therefore essential to avoid severe manifestations and complications.

Treatment of malaria in pregnancy

There is no consensus on the treatment and prophylactic drugs that a pregnant woman can and can't take. Each case must be judged on individual circumstances and risks weighed.

Treatment of malaria must not be withheld during pregnancy and pregnant women in endemic areas should be protected by chemoprophylaxis for at least the first three months of pregnancy.

Although high doses of quinine may stimulate the pregnant uterus and have been used to induce abortion, normal therapeutic doses can be used with confidence during the initial treatment of pregnant women, even in the third trimester.

Monitoring blood glucose

Monitoring of blood glucose by repeated finger-prick testing with indicator sticks is essential in pregnant women with malaria, especially if they are receiving intravenous doses of quinine, as they are more likely than other adults to develop hypoglycaemia or shortage of blood sugar. If they are at all able to eat or drink, it is preferable to try quinine by capsule or tablet rather than through a drip.

Falciparum malaria in the third trimester in non-immune women has a poor prognosis. Fever and hypoglycaemia in the mother may cause fetal distress. As the lives of the mother and fetus may be at risk, obstetrical advice should be obtained about possible induction of labour, the speeding up of the second stage of labour with forceps or a vacuum extractor, and even Caesarean section.

Antimalarial chemotherapy for pregnant women

There is general agreement that prophylaxis during pregnancy is an effective strategy. The pregnant woman should find out which drugs are safe and work best in her region and be alert for changes in their effectiveness. She must also know the possible consequences of malaria and what to do if symptoms develop.

Either rapid treatment of acute infection or effective prophylaxis is therefore essential to avoid severe manifestations and complications. (See also page 49.)

Chloroquine and quinine

Chloroquine and quinine have proved to be safe when used in normal therapeutic doses during pregnancy, and chloroquine may also be used prophylactically where it is effective.

Mefloquine (Lariam)

During the first 12–14 weeks of pregnancy, mefloquine (Lariam) should be administered for treatment only when the benefit to the mother outweighs the risk to the fetus. Until more definite results have been obtained, mefloquine prophylaxis should be avoided during pregnancy.

Proguanil (Paludrine), chlorproguanil (Lapudrine) and dapsone-pyrimethamine (Maloprim)

The use of proguanil (Paludrine), chlorproguanil (Lapudrine) and dapsone-pyrimethamine (Maloprim) to prevent malaria in pregnant women continues in some countries. However, malarial resistance to these drugs does occur. Dapsone-pyrimethamine (Maloprim) should be avoided in the third trimester of pregnancy. If used during the first two trimesters a folic acid supplement is recommended.

Doxycycline (Vibramycin)

Doxycycline (Vibramycin) is contra-indicated in pregnant women and in breastfeeding mothers.

Treatment of an acute malarial attack in pregnancy

A safe, universally acceptable treatment for malaria in pregnancy is not available. This is because all the treatment drugs carry the risk of certain side effects depending on the individual's constitution. However the following drugs have been used successfully.

Chloroquine

Chloroquine is considered safe in pregnancy. The most common adverse reaction to chloroquine is skin itching but this is encountered only in some individuals, especially black people. (See also page 94.)

Sulfadoxine-pyrimethamine (Fansidar)

Fansidar is an effective drug for treating malaria in pregnant women.

Quinine

Quinine can be given orally to pregnant women who have malaria without complications and who fail to respond to other treatment, or when other treatment is unsuitable. Both malaria and the administration of quinine can cause increased insulin production leading to hypoglycaemia. The risk of quinine producing premature labour or abortion is probably exaggerated. Quinine should not be withheld from a women with severe malaria or malaria with complications because she is pregnant.

Mefloquine (Lariam/Mephoquin)

Mefloquine is given to pregnant women, particularly in South East Asia although its safety in pregnancy has not been completely proven. The WHO does not recommend its use during pregnancy.

Halofantrine (Halfan)

Its safety and toxicity in pregnancy are not known. The manufacturers have found it to be toxic to the embryo though not implicated in the causing of deformities and have suggested that it not be used in pregnancy unless the benefits outweigh the risks. If possible, it should not be used in the first trimester.

Chemoprophylaxis, treatment and sterility

No specific link has been established between the taking of prophylactic and treatment drugs and fertility levels among men and women. However, if you are having problems with fertility, you are advised to abstain from taking prophylaxis where possible, as well as any other drug.

14. Children — at special risk

Infants and young children can become seriously ill with malaria and are at special risk. If at all possible, they should not be taken into a malarial area. If unavoidable, then all measures possible should be taken to prevent them from being bitten by mosquitoes.

Fever in a child returning from a malarious area should be considered to be caused by malaria unless proved otherwise (according to the WHO).

Infants up to six months

When a mother is immune, a degree of immunity is conferred on the fetus from the mother across the placenta and this immunity lasts approximately three to six months. Those infants with non-immune mothers are not likely to receive any immunity.

Natural immunity passes through the mother's breast milk to some extent but this has not been quantified. Infants may still become infected with malaria but seem to be resistant to developing cerebral malaria. They do become quite anaemic however.

Even if the breast-feeding mother is taking prophylaxis herself, the amount of drug that passes through the breast milk is insufficient to bestow protection. It is therefore recommended that prophylaxis be given to breast-fed and bottle-fed infants.

Chloroquine is an exception to the above as it does pass through the breast milk and if an infant is to be given chloroquine itself, it has been suggested that dosages be modified as follows:

✧ Fully breast-fed infants (four or more feeds per day) should be given half the recommended dose of chloroquine.
✧ Partially breast-fed infants (fewer than four feeds per day plus supplementary diets) should be given the full recommended paediatric dose of chloroquine.

Seven months to five years

This is the most vulnerable period in a child's life when living in an endemic area on a long term basis. The child can be compared in terms of susceptibility with a traveller who visits the area for the first time.

The child has to build up its own immunity and this is acquired over a long period of time during which the child keeps on getting bitten, and slowly raises its immunity.

The problem is that at the time of the first attack, which is likely to be the worst, the child still has minimal defences and is liable to die very quickly. Rapid diagnosis and treatment is of the utmost importance.

Attacks in endemic areas usually peak at about the age of two. Enlargement of the spleen often occurs as a result.

Six to 18 years

By now a child living in an endemic area has built up a healthy immunity to malaria. Of course, infection by a parasite to which he is not immune can still cause severe illness and even death.

Note that a child in this age group, and indeed an adult, who arrives in an endemic area for the first time, is just as vulnerable as an infant or toddler and has to go through the same process of frequent bites over a reasonably long period in order to acquire immunity.

It is worth investigating which treatment drugs will work in the endemic area you will be visiting or living in (such drugs are not yet available in suppository form).

It is not known why certain people, having lived in an endemic area for years, without taking prophylaxis, and without even getting malaria, finally get it, and get it very severely.

Table 4: Advice to be given by prescribers to the parents

1. Children are at special risk since they can rapidly become seriously ill with malaria.

2. Do not take babies or young children to a malarious area unless absolutely necessary.

3. Protect children against mosquito bites. Mosquito nets for cots and small beds are available. Keep babies under mosquito nets between dusk and dawn.

4. Give prophylaxis to breast-fed as well as to bottle-fed babies, since they are not protected by the mother's prophylaxis.

5. Chloroquine and proguanil (Paludrine) may be given safely to babies and young children. For administration, drugs may be crushed and mixed with jam.

6. Calculate the antimalarial dose as a fraction of the adult dose based on the age or weight of the child.

7. Do not give sulfadoxine-pyrimethamine (Fansidar) or sulfalene-pyrimethamine or pyrimethamine and chloroquine (Daraclor) to babies under two months of age.

8. Do not give doxycycline (Vibramycin) prophylaxis to children under eight years.

9. Mefloquine (Lariam) should not be given to children of less than 15 kg.

10. Keep all antimalarial drugs out of the reach of children and store in childproof containers. Chloroquine is particularly toxic to children if the recommended dose is exceeded.

11. Seek medical help immediately if a child develops a febrile (fever) illness. The symptoms of malaria in children may not be typical and so malaria should *always* be suspected. In babies less than three months old, malaria should be suspected even in non-febrile illness.

(Extracted from the WHO *International Travel and Health — Vaccination Requirements and Health Advice*)

Symptoms in children

Confusingly, many children with very high parasite densities in the bloodstream often display fairly mild symptoms. Therefore the slightest suspicion of malaria should be regarded in a serious light and efforts should be made to have the child's blood tested for diagnosis.

In children the manifestations are often atypical and may be alarming. Paroxysms of fever are less common, while headache, nausea, vomiting, abdominal pain, diarrhoea, a sustained fever and convulsions make up a much less characteristic clinical picture.

Cerebral malaria in children

Despite optimal care, between 10–30 per cent of children with cerebral malaria die.

This condition is frequently the only manifestation of severe *falciparum* infection in children. Convulsions form part of the symptoms of cerebral malaria.

Diagnosis

P. falciparum is usually very severe in children from non-endemic areas; diagnosis may be difficult, for parasites may not be found easily, and multiple blood smears should be taken if the first are negative. If the child is on prophylaxis and the blood smear is negative, a carefully balanced judgement, taking into account the type of prophylaxis being taken, active strains in the area and severity of illness, should be made before deciding to treat for malaria.

The incubation period is usually from six to 15 days and there are no distinctive signs in this period that the child may have contracted malaria. The first signs that he may have malaria are listlessness, restlessness and drowsiness; he may refuse food and there may be headaches or nausea. Fever is usual but variable and irregular; a regular fever cycle is uncommon and therefore not reliable as a symptom of malaria.Diarrhoea may occur and a dry cough is common. The spleen enlarges and is tender, but diagnosis should not depend on this.

Some children in highly endemic areas acquire a relative tolerance to the infection and suffer only a mild illness. Many children in such areas have large livers and spleens and malaria parasites in the blood, but no other signs of the disease.

How much time do you have with children?

Life-threatening complications may develop very rapidly in children with malaria. That is why time is so important in the treatment of malaria.In children the interval between the onset of symptoms and death may be about 48 hours, although cases have occurred where death results after only a few hours.

Chemoprophylaxis

A distinction must be made between residents of an endemic area who will live there all their lives, and those such as expatriates who eventually intend leaving the area.

Chemoprophylaxis is strongly indicated for non-local children who have not had frequent exposure to bites over a long period. It has not been established what effect long term prophylaxis will have on a child's development.

Ideally, the child should be given prophylaxis for the first few years after arrival in an endemic area, while allowing him to get bitten frequently by mosquitoes in order to acquire immunity.

It is important to remember that if a child is taken out of the endemic area for a length of time, say for a three month holiday, his levels of immunity will drop during the time he is away and his vulnerability will be increased when he returns to the endemic area. This is because immunity is dependent on frequent exposure to mosquito bites and infection.

Chloroquine and *proguanil (Paludrine)* may be safely given to babies and young children.

Pyrimethamine and *chloroquine (Daraclor)* should not be given to infants younger than six weeks.

Doxycycline (Vibramycin) is not recommended for children under eight years.

Mefloquine (Lariam) should not be given to children of less than 15 kg.

Dapsone-pyrimethamine (Maloprim) is not for use in children younger than six weeks. If used, administer Maloprim syrup in children under five years as it is not possible to break tablets into quarters.

Administration of antimalarials to infants and children

The administration of a bitter drug like chloroquine to young children is always difficult and there is no evidence that syrups are easier to administer than tablets crushed and mixed with water, jam or condensed milk. It may help to control spillage if a 5 ml syringe is used to administer the drug.

Force is often necessary (including closing the child's nostrils to make him open his mouth). There is a risk of inhalation of the medicine. A certain quantity of the drug may be spat out, leading to underdosage — or even to overdosage if repeated attempts are made to administer the drug.

While children who have received prophylaxis may have lower levels of immunity and specific antibodies, their infections are less severe clinically than those of children who have not received prophylaxis.

Most studies suggest that as suppression of malaria by prophylaxis is never complete, exposure to parasites while under the relative protection of prophylaxis might stimulate the immune system to help maintain some level of actively acquired immunity.

Suggested course of treatment if malaria is suspected in a child

Paracetamol and liquids for children needing oral rehydration are administered immediately, and the skin is cooled with tepid water and by fanning. After that a blood smear should be taken if possible. The result should be available in 10–30 minutes.

The child may by then be fit enough to take oral chloroquine if that is needed. If the child is not able to take medication by mouth he would have to be admitted to hospital and put on a drip.

Complications in the treatment of children

Vomiting may complicate the treatment of malaria, especially in children. Vomiting associated with high fever is frequently an indication for intravenous therapy, but experience shows that in a substantial proportion of children with fever, oral therapy will be possible within one or two hours after reduction of fever. (See also Chapter 12: Complications of malaria)

The long-term consequences of malaria

Repeated malaria leads to severe anaemia which increases vulnerability to other diseases and hampers development. Of course, severe anaemia itself can quickly lead to death.

15. Cerebral malaria

Cerebral malaria can be defined as a state of altered consciousness in a patient who has *P. falciparum* parasites in the blood and in whom no other cause of altered consciousness can be found (according to the WHO). In children cerebral malaria is frequently the only manifestation of severe *falciparum* malaria. Other strains of malaria, i.e. *ovale, malariae* and *vivax,* do not cause cerebral malaria.

It is not proven, but the symptoms are attributed to infected red cells clogging the inner lining of the capillaries of the brain. These infected red cells tend to become sticky and less flexible, causing a plugging or blocking effect, thus reducing the flow of the circulation.

It is not known whether cerebral malaria is caused by a certain type of parasite only, or whether it is just a heavier concentration of malarial parasites in the blood and tissues which leads to cerebral malaria, or indeed, whether only certain individuals are susceptible to it.

Diagnosis

Confusingly, many patients with cerebral malaria have scanty parasite counts and many children with very high parasite densities have fairly mild symptoms.

The longer the illness or resultant coma, the more likely the patient is to die or develop neurological consequences, a wide range of which have been observed. These include cortical blindness, blindness on one side, motor disorders, spasticity and severe mental impairment.

A lumbar puncture is essential to exclude meningitis or subarachnoid haemorrhage. In cerebral malaria the spinal fluid is usually normal, or at the most, shows only a slight rise in protein or blood cells.

Symptoms

Adults with malaria commonly have problems in other organs, usually the lungs and kidneys.

Cerebral malaria develops very rapidly. Levels of consciousness can vary from mild confusion to deep coma.

The rapidity of the descent into unconsciousness and in survivors of the emergence into full awareness are unique, distinguishing and intriguing features of cerebral malaria.

The illness may start with increasing headache, restlessness or even bizarre behaviour in rare cases. A generalised convulsion is often followed by increasing drowsiness leading to stupor and coma.

Patients with cerebral malaria often have a shortage of blood sugar or glucose. Since this is important for the brain to function, the low sugar level may worsen an already poorly functioning brain.

In adults (except those with a history of epilepsy), convulsions are a sign of cerebral malaria. Convulsing carries a real risk of inhalation of stomach contents or vomit. This is an under-recorded cause of death in cerebral malaria.

Treatment

Treatment drugs of first choice are intravenous quinine or quinidine.

Prophylactic administration of phenobarbitone decreases the number of subsequent convulsions in adults and children with cerebral malaria who are already prone to convulsions.

Measures to reduce the likelihood of convulsions and their consequences should be rigorously applied: the temperature of children should be kept as close to normal as possible by sponging with tepid water and fanning and the regular, rather than intermittent, use of paracetamol.

Patients suffering from advanced cerebral malaria require the highest level of nursing care available as they are unconscious and liable to convulsions, vomiting, aspiration pneumonia and the complications of prolonged immobility.

Prognosis

The majority of those dying from cerebral malaria are children under the age of five. The acute inflammation caused by cerebral malaria accounts for over 80 per cent of deaths from malaria. Between 10 and 50 per cent of people with cerebral malaria die. Survival depends on the level of care available and the age of the patient among other things.

In those who survive, particularly children, recovery is surprisingly rapid. More than half recover in less than 24 hours while the rest recover in 24 to 48 hours.

The prognosis for cerebral malaria is positive provided treatment is timely, apt and rapid. If the patient is reached before too much damage is done to the brain, then recovery will take place within 48 hours. It is however not uncommon for those who do recover from cerebral malaria to suffer from some type of neurological defect, although some people recover without any negative long-lasting effects.

16. Recurring malaria

Malaria may recur months to years after apparently successful treatment. In patients infected with *P. vivax* and *P. ovale*, this phenomenon is known as relapse.

Relapse is caused by dormant liver stage forms of the parasite that resume their development cycle and release merozoites into the bloodstream.

The difference between relapse and recrudescence

It is a common misconception that all types of malaria are liable to relapse. This is not true as *P. falciparum* will only recrudesce if treated incorrectly or insufficiently and the period of recurrence is limited to under a year, while the other types of malaria will cause relapse even if they are "cured".

The recurrence of malaria caused by *P. falciparum* and *P. malariae* is due to a break-out caused by surviving blood-stage parasites from an earlier infection. In the case of *P. falciparum*, break-outs usually occur within a matter of weeks rather than months. In the other strains, recurrence can be interrupted by long periods of dormancy of the parasite.

P. falciparum infections will not recur provided that prophylactic and treatment dosages have been taken correctly as prescribed (taking into account possible resistance) and provided that the strain of parasite is sensitive to the prophylactic used.

In untreated or inadequately treated malaria the parasites may persist in the body for months or years.

After the early period of recurring fever (overt malaria), the parasites are more or less in equilibrium with the forces of immunity. It is not known what triggers the sudden increase in growth in the parasites.

P. vivax malaria is characterised by a tendency to relapse from the dormant liver stage and, even if a suitable prophylactic drug has been taken regularly and continued for one month after the last risk of exposure to infection, such relapses may occur (unless a course of primaquine has been taken) and have been known to do so up to 13 months after the prophylactic was stopped.

This may cause difficulty in diagnosis. It is recommended that anti-relapse treatment of *P. vivax* infections with primaquine should be limited to two categories of patients; those living in areas where there is no *vivax* present or areas with very low levels of transmission, and those leaving the malarious area.

It is not necessary to provide anti-relapse treatment routinely to a patient living in an endemic area; in case of relapse or re-infection, such patients should be treated with an effective drug such as chloroquine.

17. Chronic malaria

The term "chronic" is applied to repeated re-infections as a result of either inadequate prophylaxis or treatment.

Chronic malaria causes progressive enlargement of the spleen, which acts as a blood cleansing organ and supplier of malaria antibodies. It is overtaxed in those who have suffered regular malaria attacks and hence becomes enlarged. This is particularly noticeable in children.

In some adults who are infected with malaria the body seems to lose control over the spleen, which continues to enlarge and eventually becomes extremely large. This condition often requires long-term antimalarial treatment. Surgical removal of the spleen is not advised.

The liver also becomes enlarged and firm, and biochemical tests may reveal a certain amount of liver dysfunction.

Children who suffer from frequent attacks of malaria do not thrive. These repeated malaria attacks deplete the body as well as produce anaemia which further weakens the system. Malaria is probably a causative factor of stunted growth.

18. Mixed infections

Mixed infections are fairly common and result when two mosquitoes carrying two different strains of the malaria parasite bite a person within a short space of time. It is also possible that one mosquito can carry two different parasites and infect the victim with both when taking its blood-feed.

Thus two different infections develop independently. During diagnosis with blood smears the technician is more likely to notice the dominant infection and therefore reporting of mixed infections is not as common as it might be.

The possibility of whether a mixed infection compounds the illness has not been well studied.

In terms of treatment, it is thought that medication taken to treat one of the strains of parasite will be effective in treating the other. Routine therapy should be followed by a 14 day course of primaquine.

A mixed infection of *vivax* and *ovale* may cause later relapses.

19. How immunity affects your response to malaria

The definition of immunity

Immunity may be natural or acquired, and complete or partial. Over many centuries those who were highly vulnerable to malaria died off, while the surviving members of the population were naturally selected from stock which possessed a high natural immunity to the disease.

Some Africans possess an inherited trait which also protects them from malaria: in this condition, called sickle cell anaemia, the haemoglobin is abnormal.

Generally, human immunity to the disease results from a capacity, following ancestral exposure to malaria, to produce proteins which specifically neutralise the harmful effects of the infecting organism. Of the two types of immunity — natural immunity (genetic/inherited) or acquired immunity, neither gives complete protection against attacks.

The eradication of mosquitoes and the loss of immunity

Ironically, it appears that the eradication of mosquitoes from a malarial area might in the long run backfire on the immune inhabitants. In time they would inevitably lose their immunity and the chance reintroduction of infected mosquitoes to their countries from another area would result in devastating epidemics.

Pregnancy and immunity

In pregnancy, a degree of immunity from the already immune mother is transferred via the placenta, causing the infant to remain immune for the first three to six months of life.

Differing degrees of immunity

It is thought that immunity may come in different degrees, for example, delay in development of the infection, mild parasitaemia (parasite counts) and complete resistance.

How immunity is built up

Immunity is built up slowly and over time. It is acquired by repeated bites from malaria-carrying mosquitoes.

A person acquires his own immunity to malaria when he has been living in a malaria endemic area for a fair length of time, a period which is closely related to the amount of exposure he has had to the bites of infected mosquitoes. For instance, a person spending five years in a malarial area who does not get bitten at all by an infected mosquito, will have no immunity whereas a person living there for a year who is constantly bitten by infected mosquitoes will be immune. During this time they should not spend any appreciable length of time out of the area as they might risk losing any immunity already acquired.

Each time a person develops full-blown malaria a certain amount of resistance develops.

It is not known exactly why a person does not get full- blown malaria each time he is bitten by an infected mosquito. It is thought that each dose is small enough for the body's immune system to cope with and overcome, but this is not proven.

Immunity is partial where malaria is seasonal but almost complete in individuals living in regions where malaria occurs all year round.

If you judiciously avoid getting bitten, it will mean that you are not exposed to any form of malaria. Your immunity level will be nil, the same as a first-time visitor to the area.

Immunity and prophylaxis

Although this issue has not been researched, it seems logical to build up an immunity by taking prophylaxis and still allowing oneself to get bitten. As no prophylactic is 100 per cent effective, a certain amount of infection with parasites will take place, hopefully little enough for the body to cope with while boosting its immune system. In the meantime the prophylactic should afford a reasonably large measure of protection against developing full-blown malaria.

Specific immunity

If the period of ill-health in childhood is successfully negotiated, a balance is achieved between infection and resistance.

Resistance is developed against the specific strain of malaria a person is most exposed to. Therefore, if you move to a different part of the country and are infected by a different strain there, your immune system may not be able to recognise and fight that particular strain.

Types of immunity

There are three classes of immunity:

- ✧ *non-immune* e.g. travellers, young children, military personnel, refugees, tourists and those in whom established immunity has lapsed, pregnant women, who are more vulnerable, inhabitants of an endemic area who leave and then return and residents of an area where a successful malaria control programme has been concluded.
- ✧ *partially or semi-immune* e.g. those who live in areas where transmission of malaria is irregular, e.g. only during the rainy season; or those who spend a fair amount of time outside their country of residence where transmission is year-round.
- ✧ *fully immune* e.g. those who live continually in a country where malaria transmission is year-round and who have lived their childhood years in the same place.

Non-immune

If travel to malarious areas is unavoidable, travellers should obtain, before departure, the addresses of reliable medical services at their destination. They should also make certain that they are covered by insurance for emergency evacuation to their home country.

If the traveller is likely to be hypersensitive to an antimalarial drug or is taking other drugs for long-term medical conditions, he should consult a doctor with specialised knowledge of the problem before departure and decide whether his journey is essential.

The traveller who is lacking a spleen, has problems with his immune system or suffers from diseases such as lymphoma, cardiac conditions, leukaemia (even in remission) or Hodgkin's disease should make prior arrangements for adequate medical care at his destination and should seek this care immediately if he should fall ill.

It is generally recommended that women who are pregnant should not travel to malarious areas (see section on pregnancy, page 54). Pregnant women, and children under five, are most vulnerable to contracting malaria. During pregnancy the immune system is not at its best. Expectant mothers exposed to malaria are most vulnerable during first or second pregnancies and in the first trimester.

As the malignant malaria (*P. falciparum)* parasites take between six and 14 days to incubate, and those parasites responsible for the more benign forms (mainly *P. vivax*) may take much longer to incubate, a disease that starts before six days have elapsed since the first exposure is probably not malaria.

Early diagnosis and prompt treatment are the most vital survival tools for those who may have malignant malaria. A non-immune person who develops fever six days or more after the first possible exposure to malaria should seek prompt medical attention while informing the doctor that he may have malaria.

Most travellers who contract malaria initially develop the disease without complications although the progression to severe anaemia is usually very rapid.

The choice of drug treatment for travellers (see Appendix, page 90) depends, as it does with all malaria patients, on the species of malaria parasite prevalent where the infection was contracted. Parasite sensitivities to antimalarial drugs vary greatly around the world (see page 11).

Depending on the country visited, the appropriate drugs and prompt medical attention may not be available. Non-immune travellers are advised to carry certain antimalarial drugs as standby treatment. This stand-by treatment may be used as self-treatment but, preferably, should be used only after obtaining medical advice.

Because of the possibility of toxic reactions, travellers should resort to self-treatment only if they have good reason to suspect malaria and prompt medical attention is not available.

Medical attention should be sought at the earliest possible opportunity and the doctor should be told which drugs were taken and in what dosages. If possible keep a close watch on symptoms and note them down so that you can inform the doctor of the progression of the disease.

The typical symptoms of malaria are bouts of high fever lasting a few hours, beginning with shaking chills, subsiding with profuse sweating, and recurring at regular intervals, usually every 48 hours.

It is worth noting that the signs are often atypical during the first few days and are less typical in malignant than in benign malaria.

Therefore the possibility of malaria should be considered in all otherwise unexplained fevers in non-immune persons who have been exposed to mosquitoes.

Partially immune

Partial immunity develops over time through repeated infection and without recurrent infection. Immunity is relatively short-lived when malaria transmission is not ongoing in the country of residence or when the person has spent lengthy periods of time out of his country of residence, thereby losing any immunity he may have gained.

People with partial immunity are as vulnerable as those with no immunity at all, as they are not able to rely on their immunity status for protection.

Fully immune

There really is no such thing as a person who is fully immune to malaria. He may be almost completely immune to one or two strains of parasite but because of geographical variations in the distributions of the various strains of malaria parasite, he may not be immune to strains prevalent in areas which he rarely visits.

Immune individuals produce antibodies capable of binding specifically to the infected red cell surface, thereby facilitating their destruction by splenic and other cells.

Fully immune people have lived in an area with year-round malaria transmission for a very long time, or they have an inherited tendency to overcome malaria.

If and when they do get malaria, it is generally not severe, although there are of course some cases that are, and the individual is usually able to overcome the infection on his own. There may be fever or vague complaints of headache, body pains or a general malaise.

Without repeated exposure however, this immunity is relatively short-lived and although it almost always protects against life-threatening malaria, it does not prevent occasional bouts of fever and chills.

Researchers postulate that some people tolerate malaria infections without symptoms whereas others are severely affected because they have become desensitised to the breakdown products formed by the parasite.

There can be little doubt that when given extremely conscientiously, malaria prophylaxis will interfere with the development of malaria immunity, for example, in expatriates resident in malaria endemic areas.

When prophylaxis is not conscientious, occasional breakthrough infections occur which may be as effective at inducing protective immunity as repeated and heavy exposure. (See page 107 on whether to give prophylaxis or not.)

Prevention of relapses

The drugs recommended for prophylaxis, with the possible exceptions of proguanil (Paludrine) and doxycycline (Vibramycin), do not eliminate the liver stages of relapsing malaria infections, i.e. *P. vivax* in most of the malarious areas and *P. ovale* in West Africa.

The liver stages can lead to relapses up to three years after exposure, but these relapses are not life-threatening.

They can be prevented by primaquine; an anti-relapse course of primaquine may be considered for persons who have been exposed to a relatively high risk for six months or more. Primaquine should be taken only under medical supervision.

20. How can you avoid getting malaria?

Medical consensus on the whole suggests that the prevention of mosquito bites is the main form of protection against malaria as no drug is 100 per cent effective. Chemical protection by means of drugs is only a secondary alternative.

In addition, protection largely depends on the individual's motivation to seek useful advice and act upon it. It depends on the perception of the risk to which the person is exposed and the severity of malaria. The individual must also understand the types of protective measures that are at his disposal and his need to comply with these measures.

Most of the above conditions may be met, but if coupled with less than perfect compliance, especially with chemoprophylactic measures, then protection may be reduced significantly.

Among travellers in particular, reasons for non-compliance include forgetfulness, especially by those who travel often and have busy schedules; inadequate information and time for preparation prior to departure; confusion from contradictory information; unpleasant side effects of the drug or other illness; or that recommended protective measures are complicated.

Those travelling to endemic areas where drug resistance is experienced, should be made aware of the type of symptoms which may develop despite taking antimalarial drugs, and that may well indicate a malaria infection. They should realise that symptoms can become apparent while they are still in the area or even after they have stopped taking prophylaxis up to a period of three months after their return. They must also know what to do in the event that they experience symptoms.

Protection through the use of prophylactic drugs should be individualised. The following factors should be taken into account before deciding whether to take prophylaxis or not, and if taken, what kind of protective measures should be taken.

◇ Prevalence of mosquitoes in area visited
   − Is it situated at high or low altitude? (urban or rural)
   − Is the area visited likely to be in city centres and air-conditioned buildings?
   − Is the visit during the dry or wet season?
◇ Incidence of the parasite's resistance to the drug will determine which drugs are more likely to confer protection
◇ Purpose of visit (e.g. business or safari)
◇ Type of accommodation available (i.e. screened or air-conditioned)
◇ Duration of stay in the area — the longer the visit, the greater the risk of contracting malaria. Another risk to be taken into account is the longer the need to take a drug, the greater the risk of potential side effects.
◇ Time of year (is transmission steady throughout the year or are there peak periods of transmission?)
◇ Availability of the drug
◇ Toxicity of available drugs
◇ Age of patient, which will determine drug selection and dosage as well as vulnerability to malaria
◇ Pregnancy or lactation
◇ Immune status
◇ Medical facilities and their availability and adequacy
◇ Drug allergies
◇ Concurrent medication
◇ Use of protective measures, their efficacy and compliance with them.

No prophylactic regimen can be expected to give perfect protection. To complicate matters, most drugs used for prophylaxis are associated with some toxic side effects.

The WHO points out that it is no longer true that prophylaxis is always better than no prophylaxis, nor is it true that a more effective but less safe drug is always preferable to a less effective but safer one.

Whatever approach is taken, it is essential that it be backed up by prompt diagnosis and treatment of malaria.

In the light of the conditional nature of the risk of malaria and the issue of prophylaxis, the elderly, the very young, and pregnant women should consider very carefully whether travel to malarious areas is unavoidable. Other persons at high risk who should avoid a malarious area altogether are individuals whose immune systems are compromised i.e. those who have been on long-term steroid therapy; cancer patients on chemotherapy; AIDS patients; and those who have had their spleens removed.

Measures that prevent infection involve personal protection against bites with mosquito coils, vapours, sprays and nets.

The only measure for protecting against disease without preventing infection would be immunisation, an option that will not be available to us for a long time yet.

21. Mechanical protection

International Travel and Health — Vaccination Requirements and Health Advice, published by the WHO, includes the following guidelines:

✧ If available, choose screened or airconditioned accommodation (remembering that doors to such accommodation should be kept closed unless they are screened, to prevent the daytime entry of mosquitoes).

✧ Where this is not available, make effective use of a mosquito net preferably impregnated with insecticide.

✧ Use long-sleeved clothing and trousers when outdoors in the evening; keep the ankles protected as much as possible.

✧ Apply a mosquito repellent to exposed skin (while taking note of manufacturer's recommendations, especially for young children).

✧ Where screened sleeping accommodation is available, clear the room of any resting mosquitoes by using an insecticide aerosol, preferably a synthetic pyrethroid.

✧ Where electricity is available, plug in insecticide dispensers using mats impregnated with synthetic pyrethroid. They are a compact and useful addition to the traveller's kit.

✧ Don't go outside at night if you can avoid it. Bear in mind that large numbers of indigenous children are usually carriers of malaria parasites: avoid staying nearby if possible.

✧ Don't allow children to play in dark shady areas. Avoid places with banana, sisal and maize plantations nearby as they may provide resting sites for mosquitoes.

✧ Where safe sprays are available, it is advisable to spray the internal walls of houses every three months.

✧ All ventilation holes should be screened to prevent insects from coming through them.

✧ Make sure there are no containers of water exposed for mosquitoes to breed in.

✧ Insecticide-impregnated mosquito nets have proved to be almost totally effective, but they must be scrupulously maintained to avoid tearing. There should be no opening on the side of the net, which ideally should be lowered and tucked well in under the mattress before dusk and not raised until after dawn. Mosquitoes will enter a torn or sloppily used net, which then becomes a mosquito trap.

✧ Long term residents in malarious areas should, if they can, situate houses 1 km or more away from water points or streams; hill tops are usually better than valleys. The windows of houses should be covered by a special metal gauze manufactured for the purpose. Mosquito-proof screen doors may be added to outside doors so that they can be kept open to allow maximum air movement inside without letting mosquitoes in.

✧ Mosquitoes tend to lurk under tables and chairs and the ankles are therefore particularly vulnerable to bites. Two pairs of stockings are not enough to prevent bites.

✧ When spraying a room, pay particular attention to dark corners, spaces beneath chairs and tables and also to wardrobes, cupboards, bathrooms and lavatories.

22. Questions commonly asked about malaria

Are the following statements true?

✧ If you habitually drink gin and tonic you are less likely to get malaria. (Answer: The level of quinine in the tonic is thought to be too low to prevent malaria.)

✧ If you are bitten in the afternoon, it will not be by a mosquito carrying the malaria parasite. (Answer: It is unlikely to be by one carrying malaria.)

✧ Only the female mosquito will transmit malaria. (Answer: Yes)

✧ The malaria-carrying mosquito makes no noise. (Answer: It makes a slight noise.)

✧ If I have AIDS and get malaria, I will die from the attack. (Answer: No. AIDS does not make malaria worse.)

✧ Malaria will surface when the host's immune system is compromised. (Answer: Yes, unless there is a balance between immunity and parasite levels.)

✧ With *ovale* malaria, your body will have overcome the infection after three years. (Answer: Yes, as the parasite stops relapsing.)

✧ You can contract malaria from a blood transfusion. (Answer: Yes, if the blood has not been screened properly for malaria parasites.)

✧ Malaria can exist in cold climates such as England. (Answer: Whatever malaria exists will be short-lived and invariably brought over on an aeroplane from a malarious country. All it needs for the disease to occur is one malaria-carrying mosquito biting a few people before dying from unfavourable conditions.)

✧ There are long term effects of malaria. (Answer: Yes; anaemia results when the ongoing destruction of the blood cells by maturing malaria parasites over a period of time gradually lowers the blood count; disturbed liver function and enlarged spleen are results of ongoing parasite infection.

23. The long term outlook for malaria

Where will we stand by the year 2000?

Globally, the malaria situation is getting worse. This is mainly due to the complex nature of the malaria parasite which has enabled it to so successfully resist the numerous and varied attempts to both control it and wipe it out.

Recognising that the worldwide eradication of the disease is not an attainable goal in the foreseeable future, the WHO Expert Committee on Malaria decided that its main objective should be to provide easily accessible and appropriate diagnostic and treatment facilities for the entire population of malarious areas.

Currently there are three main possibilities, none immediately available, which may be used only as individual components in the strategy to fight malaria. These include the Chinese wonder drug artemisinin, a malaria vaccine and the much vaguer prospect of reversal of chloroquine resistance.

Artemisinin

Drug research has aroused much interest in artemisinin, a new class of antimalarial drug that has its roots in ancient Chinese history.

For some 2000 years, the leaves and flowering heads of *Artemisia annua* (the sweet wormwood plant) have been used in Chinese traditional medicine to treat fever and chills associated with malaria. Artemisinin is the active antimalarial constituent. It was isolated by Chinese scientists in 1972. The traditional medicine *qinghaosu* is derived from the same plant.

Artemisinin has marked activity against malaria parasites, including multidrug-resistant *P. falciparum*. Available in China in suppository form and in intra-muscular injection form, it should be released in the West, probably France, before 1995.

The drug and its derivatives have been used to treat thousands of patients with *falciparum* malaria in China. The results show that it is capable of rapid initial clearance of parasitaemia (about five hours only), possibly faster than any other drug, a lack of serious toxicity and in studies of severe *falciparum* malaria, exceptional efficacy. However, as infections frequently relapse it is best combined with another drug.

Artemether is shown to be powerful with apparently low toxicity. Derivatives of artemisinin have been synthesised, and some researchers cautiously express the hope that these may prove to be among the most potent weapons in the arsenal used in the fight against malaria since quinine was isolated in 1834 from the bark of the Cinchona tree.

Immunisation

Although much work has been done in the development of a vaccine, we are still many years away from the release and active use of a universally applicable vaccine.

Even once a vaccine is released, it will not provide blanket coverage of populations living in endemic areas. Rather it will be used to protect those groups most at risk.

A Colombian scientist has developed a vaccine that is said to work only on certain strains of the malaria parasite. He has offered the patent on the vaccine to the WHO and at present trials are being carried out in Kenya. At present the vaccination appears to provide a 40 per cent immunity to adults and 77 per cent to young children.

A divergent approach to the vaccine problem involves developing a vaccine for humans which would in turn vaccinate the biting mosquito, rendering it an inhospitable host for the malaria parasite.

Untreatable malaria

The most frightening prospect of all, untreatable malaria, is continuously mentioned in connection with countries in South East Asia. As we head towards the next century, new strains of malaria parasite are developing in Thailand which are resistant to all conventional drugs. The problem is exacerbated by the repatriation of some 20 000 refugees to Cambodia.

Despite the existence of so-called untreatable malaria, researchers believe that all malaria can be treated and cured, but this may now require a combination of drugs rather than relying on the administration of only one kind of drug.

Only extremely diligent management of resources used to fight malaria and strict control of drug availability will help to make any headway in the fight against malaria. Already, the WHO has admitted that they have given up the fight against malaria (WHO Conference, Amsterdam, October 1992) and that their aim now is only to control it rather than eradicate it.

Appendix 1: Treatment options

Not everyone reading this book will have to decide for themselves which drug to take for treatment or prophylaxis. However, there will be those who need to have such information at hand, merely because other information sources are not readily available or because they wish to expand on information they may already have obtained from their doctor.

Warning

It is intended that in all cases where medical help is available, the patient should attempt to obtain it and not treat himself. No responsibility will be taken by the author or publisher for any negative consequences arising out of advice taken from this book.

The most important aspects of treatment

✧ prompt and effective treatment with antimalarials
✧ correction of fluid and electrolyte substances if there has been a fluid loss
✧ correction of hypoglycaemia or low blood sugar, especially in diabetics and pregnant women
✧ correction of anaemia
✧ treatment of concurrent infection if one exists.

When to treat for malaria

If *P. falciparum* is suspected, even if test results are not yet available or are negative, if the patient has fever or any of the other signs of malaria (see page 27), antimalarial treatment must be given. If another illness is suspected at the same time, treat for that as well.

The most important aim in treatment

The most important aim in treatment is to bring the level of parasites present in the blood *under control as quickly as possible* by the administration of rapidly acting drugs. This presents little difficulty except in *P. falciparum* malaria, where the progression of the disease is extremely rapid.

The different types of treatment drug available

The name in the column on the left in table 5 is the generic name, commonly used by doctors and medical personnel. The names on the right are the trade names which are likely to be more familiar to the public.

This is an area of potentially major confusion, when one drug is given more than one trade name or when patients do not understand to which drug their doctor is referring.

Trade names also differ in different countries. Some treatment drugs are used as prophylactics while others are used exclusively for treatment, yet others are used for both.

Table 5: Malaria drugs

Treatment only	
Amodiaquine:*	Camoquin, Flavoquine or Basoquin
Halofantrine:	Halfan
Primaquine:	Primaquine
Quinine:	Quinine
Sulfadoxine-pyrimethamine:	Fansidar
Prophylaxis and treatment (see also page 107)	
Chloroquine-phosphate:	Aralen, Avloclor, Delagil, Lagaquin, Lariago, Malaviron, Resochin, Starquine
Chloroquine-sulph:	Nivaquine
Hydroxychloroquine-sulph:	Plaguenil (not often used for malaria, more for rheumatoid arthritis)

Mefloquine:	Mephaquin, Lariam

Prophylaxis only

Doxycycline:	Vibramycin
Dapsone-pyrimethamine:	Maloprim
Proguanil:	Paludrine, Paludrinol
Pyrimethamine:	Daraprim, Tindurin
Sulphametopyrazine-pyrimethamine:	Metakelfin
Chlorproguanil:	Lapudrine

* This drug is no longer recommended for use by the WHO.

Chloroquine

This long-time stand-by is used to treat chloroquine-sensitive *P. falciparum* or *P. malariae* and to terminate acute attacks of *P. vivax* or *P. ovale* malaria.

The tablets usually contain 150 mg of chloroquine base per tablet. For a malaria attack, a total course of treatment would comprise 25 mg/kg, usually given orally in a three day course for the treatment of chloroquine-sensitive *P. falciparum*.

The standard regimen consists of 10 mg base per kg of body weight followed by 5 mg/kg six to eight hours later and 5 mg/kg on each of the second and third days (WHO *Practical Chemotherapy of Malaria*). To eliminate the risk of nausea and vomiting, do not take on an empty stomach.

Table 6 gives the total amount of chloroquine to be taken over three days according to body weight.

Table 6: Chloroquine dosages

5 kg	125 mg	just under 1/2 tablet
10 kg	250 mg	just over 3/4 tablet
15 kg	375 mg	one tablet and 1/4
20 kg	500 mg	one tablet and 2/3
30 kg	750 mg	two tablets and 1/2
40 kg	1 000 mg	three tablets and 1/3

50 kg	1 250 mg	four tablets and under 1/4
60 kg	1 500 mg	five tablets
70 kg	1 750 mg	five tablets and over 3/4
80 kg	2 000 mg	six tablets and 2/3
90 kg	2 250 mg	seven tablets and 1/2
100 kg	2 500 mg	eight tablets and 1/3
110 kg	2 750 mg	nine tablets

Chloroquine resistance

Resistance to chloroquine by the malaria parasite (*P. falciparum*) has spread to most areas of the world except the Middle East, Central America, and the Caribbean. Estimated resistance is usually expressed as a percentage. If there is 60 per cent chloroquine resistance in an area, chloroquine may still be used as the drug of choice. If there is 80 per cent resistance, then chloroquine will not be used and Fansidar or another drug will, more likely, be used in its place.

Recent reports of resistance to chloroquine by *P. vivax* have been received.

Resistance to chloroquine is present throughout the area of distribution of *P. falciparum* in South-east Asia. Chloroquine has lost practically all its therapeutic effect in Thailand and some parts of Myanmar (formerly Burma).

Resistance to sulfadoxine-pyrimethamine (Fansidar) combination (SP) has also developed in vast areas of Thailand, some parts of Myanmar, Bangladesh, Bhutan and Indonesia. (See untreatable malaria in previous chapter, and list of countries where chloroquine is no longer effective, page 11.)

Prior to the surge of resistance, the continuation of fever for roughly 24 to 32 hours after treatment by chloroquine meant that the patient was ill from another cause. Now it probably means that the chloroquine has failed to do its job because of resistance. The problem lies in the fact that while chloroquine is not doing the job it is supposed to do, the malaria infection is growing and becoming more severe and precious time is lost in the battle against it.

Contra-indications

Chloroquine should not be used

❖ when there is high resistance to the drug
❖ when an infection has broken through despite the use of chloroquine as a prophylactic
❖ when malaria does not appear to be responding to treatment with chloroquine
❖ if there is any doubt about the origin of the infection
❖ in patients with impaired liver or kidney function, porphyria or psoriasis. Alcoholics tend to have an adverse reaction to chloroquine.

Side effects

Adverse effects are rare and mild when the drug is given orally in the usual antimalarial doses. Nausea and vomiting may occur if it is taken on an empty stomach. Headache and visual difficulties have been reported in patients receiving a therapeutic regimen of 25 mg/kg. Pruritus, or itching of palms, soles and scalp has been reported in up to 20 per cent of Africans using chloroquine, a condition that is not relieved by antihistamines.

All these symptoms are reversible upon discontinuation of the medication.

Repeated and prolonged prophylactic use of chloroquine requires that the user have eye checks every three to six months.

Symptoms of poisoning by overdosage include headache, nausea, diarrhoea, dizziness, muscular weakness and blurred vision. Severe poisoning has been treated successfully by intensive hospital care.

Amodiaquine (Camoquin)

This drug was used in areas where a high degree of chloroquine resistance was encountered. *However its use is no longer recommended anywhere by the WHO.*

In view of the risks associated with Camoquin and its limited therapeutic advantages, it should not be used for prevention of malaria or treatment either as a drug of first choice or even as a more restricted alternative for chloroquine failures.

Side effects

Like chloroquine, Camoquin causes pruritus. It also carries risks of toxic hepatitis and potentially lethal agranulocytosis (white blood cells stop being produced). It may cause severe suppression of the bone marrow when used for prophylaxis over a long time.

Quinine

Where resistance to chloroquine is encountered, quinine is usually the drug that saves. It is likely to be administered together with tetracycline where resistance to quinine alone is present.

Because of its usually unpleasant side effects and in order to slow the spread of resistance to it, quinine is used only in cases of severe malaria, usually when other treatments have failed.

Whenever severe *falciparum* malaria is encountered it is preferable that quinine be given intravenously until the infection has been brought under control. Once it has and the patient can take medication by mouth, then it is given orally.

Quinine is administered either orally or by injection. It is extremely valuable because of its rapid action on parasites. It may be combined with tetracycline, an antibiotic, or sulfadoxine-pyrimethamine (Fansidar), which by reducing the length of quinine treatment, helps reduce the quinine-related side effects.

Some resistance to quinine has developed, particularly in Thailand where it has been used extensively for malaria therapy. Whenever it is used, it should be under medical or hospital supervision.

Contra-indications

Quinine should not be used in those with a history of hypersensitivity to quinine, with heart disease, or those taking anticoagulants.

Side effects

Side effects in many patients include: giddiness, light-headedness, temporary hearing loss, tinnitus (ringing in the ears) and blurred vision.

Anorexia (loss of appetite), nausea and vomiting may occur after the first few doses although these may be difficult to distinguish from the symptoms of acute malaria.

Less frequent but more serious side effects of quinine include abnormal cardiac rhythms, thrombocytopenia (low platelet count), haemolysis (destruction of red blood cells) and oedema (increase in tissue fluids) of the eyelids, mucous membranes and lungs. These may occur following a single dose and necessitate immediate discontinuation of the drug.

Repeat administration of quinine in full therapeutic doses may give rise to a train of symptoms known as "cinchonism", characterised by tinnitus, headache, nausea, abdominal pain, pruritus, other skin rashes, disturbed vision and even temporary blindness.

Some patients are hypersensitive to quinine and even small doses may give rise to symptoms of cinchonism, asthma and other allergic phenomena.

Hypoglycaemia (low blood sugar) due to malaria may be aggravated by oral treatment of even low doses of quinine, as a result of stimulation of insulin secretion. This is a particularly important consideration in the treatment of malaria in pregnant women, whose blood glucose should be carefully monitored.

Quinine treatment has been considered dangerous in pregnancy. Recent work, however, suggests that therapeutic doses do not induce labour and that the stimulation of contractions and evidence of fetal distress associated with the use of quinine may be more properly attributed to the presence of fever and other effects of the malaria itself.

Tetracycline

This is an effective but slow blood schizontocide (meaning that it kills mature malaria parasites) in the therapy of malaria.

It is usually administered orally with the more fast-acting quinine so that initial control of parasite levels and symptoms is established. This combination has been found to be highly effective in treating infections resistant to quinine.

Tetracycline should only be given orally and should not be given to pregnant women or to children under the age of eight, except when the risk of withholding the drug outweighs the risk of damage to developing teeth or bones.

Side effects

The most common side effects of tetracycline administration are gastrointestinal, including epigastric distress, abdominal discomfort, nausea, vomiting and diarrhoea as well as phototoxicity, or extreme sensitivity to light.

Long term tetracycline administration may result in a change of the normal intestinal bacterial flora and overgrowth of the bowel with *Candida, E. coli* and pathogenic *staphylococci*. This can be offset by taking *lactobacillus acidophilus* or yoghurt tablets, usually available in health shops.

Quinidine may be used instead of quinine where quinine is unobtainable, as in the USA where it is not registered.

Sulfadoxine-pyrimethamine (Fansidar)

The drug Fansidar (sulfadoxine-pyrimethamine) is used as a first line treatment in areas of high chloroquine resistance such as Malawi and Kenya.

Even when an infection has been acquired in a fairly chloroquine-resistant part of the world, doctors may prefer to use quinine in treatment of all cases of severe *falciparum* malaria.

This is because sulfadoxine-pyrimethamine (Fansidar) is capable of producing severe adverse reactions in some people, especially those who are allergic to sulfa drugs. Severe allergic reactions may cause death.

Others who should not use Fansidar are:

✧ newborn infants
✧ pregnant women, although it may be used in late pregnancy
✧ persons with kidney or liver disorders.

Its use has been linked with bone-marrow suppression, usually with prolonged dosage. The more widespread use of Fansidar as a treatment drug in recent times has led to an increased resistance to it.

It was previously used as a prophylactic but its use was associated with the development of Stevens-Johnson Syndrome. Its main advantage over quinine is that it is administered in a single dose:

under 4 years :	1/2 tablet
4-8 years :	1 tablet
9-14 years :	2 tablets
over 14 years :	3 tablets

(Confirm with local doctor, if at all possible.)

Halofantrine (Halfan)

Halfan is indicated for treatment of acute malaria caused by single or mixed infections of *P. falciparum* or *P. vivax*.

Limited data indicate favourable results with the strains *P. ovale* and *P. malariae*.

Treatment with Halfan is contra-indicated during pregnancy unless benefits are thought to outweigh risks. Nor is its use recommended in breastfeeding mothers.

Side effects

According to the manufacturers, Halfan is generally well tolerated. Abdominal pain, diarrhoea, pruritus and skin rash have been reported but a causal relationship has not been established. It may be poorly absorbed and a second treatment, a week later, is advised.

Mefloquine (Lariam)

Related chemically to quinine, mefloquine is effective against parasites that are resistant to quinine and other drug combinations. It can be used as a treatment drug or for short-term prophylaxis of not longer than three months.

Registered in 1984, it is a comparatively new drug. It is used for treatment in a single dose.

Side effects

The main adverse reactions are dizziness, disturbed balance, nausea, vomiting, diarrhoea, abdominal pain and loss of appetite.

Effects are mild to moderate and do not require specific treatment. Severe dizziness has been reported in certain individuals.

There are reports of serious adverse neurological and psychiatric effects following both the therapeutic and prophylactic use of mefloquine. These reactions have ranged from fatigue and weakness, malaise to seizures and acute psychosis and have been reported following the use of both mefloquine alone and in fixed combination with sulfadoxine-pyrimethamine (Fansidar). Serious adverse effects are reported to have taken place after three to five weeks of prophylaxis.

Extreme caution must be exercised in the use of mefloquine in patients concurrently taking beta-blockers, calcium-channel blockers, digitalis or antidepressants until further convincing evidence is available on the interaction of mefloquine with cardioactive agents. Those who need fine motor co-ordination in the course of employment or travel should also exercise caution in its use.

Drug interaction studies between mefloquine and many other widely used drugs are not complete and therefore any patients receiving additional medication must be closely observed.

The use of mefloquine is contra-indicated for three months before conception, during pregnancy, in children weighing less than 15 kg, in those suffering from depression and in those with apparent underlying seizure disorders.

Primaquine

Primaquine is highly active against gametocytes and against the latent liver stages of relapsing malarias but has little blood (schizontocidal) activity. This means that it is more useful for treating the relapsing malarias as caused by *P. ovale* and *vivax*.

The usual dose for anti-relapse therapy of *P. vivax* and *P. ovale* is 15 mg base daily for 14 days. A course of chloroquine is usually given first to kill the acute phase of the disease.

Toxic symptoms are rare when primaquine is given at the usual dosage. Primaquine should be given with extreme care to patients being treated with myeloid depressant drugs or who suffer from bone-marrow suppression from whatever cause.

Contra-indications

Patients with a genetic deficiency of the enzyme G6PD should not be treated with primaquine. It is usual to do a blood test to detect any G6PD deficiency before treatment.

Primaquine should be avoided in pregnancy in case the fetus is G6PD-deficient.

Drug resistance defined

Resistance describes the parasite's ability to withstand the effects of a drug. This reduces the drug's ability to cure the disease. Resistance occurs under the following conditions:

◇ widespread use of the drug
◇ insufficient dosage
◇ partial administration of the course of drugs

When insufficient dosage and partial administration take place, the parasites in the bloodstream are said to be "selected" for resistance. That is, the stronger parasites that can overcome the limited effect of the drug survive to breed more of their kind, while the weaker ones which succumb to the drug, die out, leaving only resistant parasites.

The parasites will breed and sooner or later a new infection will break out and require treatment.

The next time the drug is taken its job will be much harder as it will have to fight against resistant parasites. The chances are that it will fail in its task.

Conditions requiring special care in medication

◇ *Sulfa sensitive patients* should avoid Maloprim and Fansidar.
◇ *Cardiac patients*: quinidine is more likely to cause cardiac effects such as arrhythmias and hypersensitivity reactions. There is a danger of drug interaction between mefloquine and calcium-channel blockers, beta-blockers and digitalis.

- *Patients with liver or kidney disorders* should not take tetracycline.
- *Newborn infants* should be protected against mosquito bites.
- *Pregnant women's* blood glucose must be carefully monitored for hypoglycaemia if quinine is used as treatment; do not take halofantrine or mefloquine. Do not take primaquine, because of potential damage to the fetus.
- *Lactating mothers* should not take halofantrine
- *Depressive patients* taking diazepam (anti-depressives) should not use mefloquine.
- *Those who have had repeated, frequent malaria attacks*, particularly if there is a suspicion of treatment failure, need specialised care
- *G6PD deficient patients* should not take primaquine.
- *Porphyria sufferers* should not take sulpha or sulphonamide drugs or chloroquine.

Why it is important to take the entire course of treatment

If only a proportion of the entire treatment dosage is taken, enough to kill off a sufficient number of the parasites to eliminate symptoms of the disease, but not enough to kill all the parasites in the blood, this will result in a recurrence of the malaria in a few weeks' time when the parasites have had a chance to build up to levels that overcome the body's immune system.

Another effect of not taking a sufficient dosage or the full course of treatment is that parasites are selected that are less sensitive to the drug. If these multiply, a new strain of resistant parasite, which responds less to that drug, becomes more widespread.

The hierarchy of drug defence

Here one needs to distinguish between a country's drug prescription policy and the options open to an individual.

In an area where there is resistance to chloroquine, it depends on how much reported resistance exists as to whether the first drug to be used for treatment will be chloroquine or not.

If strong resistance is reported, the drug of choice may be sulfadoxine-pyrimethamine (Fansidar) or halofantrine (Halfan). If the case is severe and complicated, quinine and tetracycline must be considered as the drug of choice.

What if it doesn't work?

It will be seen within 48 hours that symptoms have not been relieved, that the fever is still occurring at intervals and that the patient's condition is deteriorating. It is usual to retest the blood for a parasite count and then change the course of therapy. However, many factors are at play here including the parasite's sensitivity to the drug used.

What if you wait too long to treat malaria?

Unless malaria is treated immediately, symptoms will be extreme and the more complicated forms of malaria may arise: certainly there is a high risk of anaemia and cerebral malaria as well as kidney failure.

The patient must be hospitalised and treatment for the various complications given.

There is a highly significant correlation between the delay in starting treatment and death. To have any impact on a patient, chemotherapy must be started as soon as possible.

What are the consequences of self-medication?

If the right drug is used and the right dosage is given in good enough time, the chances are that the patient will recover. However, there is always a risk that the patient is given too little or too much of a drug, or that a drug is used to which the parasites are resistant.

Probably the most common and the most serious consequence of unsuccessful self-medication is delay in seeking treatment. With malaria a delay of four days can prove fatal. An average of 2.8 days between the onset of symptoms and death was found in children in The Gambia, although it is not known why some died much sooner.

The dangers of self-medication

✧ You might choose the right drug but the incorrect dosage for your body weight.

✧ The confusing range of drugs that can be taken: you might start medication with one type of tablet and switch to another if symptoms do not improve. The new drug may be just a different form of the same drug and therefore be as ineffective as the first drug. In the meantime, the malaria will have progressed and got worse.

✧ Overdosage: you might start to take a drug, not feel better, visit a doctor and omit to tell him you have taken the drug. He may give you a drug which when taken in combination with the drug you have already taken, results in overdosage or incompatibility and consequently serious side effects.

✧ Self-medication with antimalarials may be used for symptoms that are not malaria at all and other causes of fever will go undetected or untreated.

Simultaneous treatment for malaria

Rehydration

Rehydration is vital in hot climates. Patients with fever may become dehydrated very quickly, especially if they are vomiting and have diarrhoea simultaneously.

Children are especially at risk from dehydration. They are likely to be intolerant of fasting and may therefore become hypoglycaemic. Glucose supplements included in oral rehydration formulas for the control of diarrhoea may help control the hypoglycaemia.

Where vomiting or dehydration is not present, it is sufficient for cool liquids to be given. Alcoholic beverages worsen dehydration. Where vomiting or diarrhoea is present, give the commercially available, specially formulated oral rehydration therapy (ORT) powder, which is mixed with cooled boiled water. This contains salts and sugars to replace those that were lost through vomiting and diarrhoea.

If you have no access to specially formulated powders, make up your own. This consists of one teaspoon of salt and six tablespoons of sugar in one litre of cooled, boiled water (see also dehydration remedy on page 38). This is likely to be unpalatable to children who may prefer to take diluted flat Coca Cola. Never give milk or other dairy products to a person with vomiting and diarrhoea.

Bed rest and lowering of body temperature may reduce vomiting and allow patients to be treated orally. If the frequency of vomiting or diarrhoea is such that it prevents the patient from keeping down fluids and medicine, he should be hospitalised and administered liquids through a drip.

Reducing fever

Fever needs to be reduced to control the risk of convulsions, especially in young children. Typically, malaria produces high fevers of 39 °C and above.

Physical methods, such as removal of clothes, fanning and sponging with lukewarm water are the most reliable.

Various antifever drugs are used in the treatment of malaria patients. Paracetamol is preferred to aspirin and it can be given by mouth or suppository. Suppositories are indicated for infants or children, or where vomiting is preventing the absorption of the drug. Crushed tablets can be administered via nasogastric tube.

Combating anaemia

As more and more red blood cells are destroyed by the malaria parasites, the blood's oxygen-carrying capacity decreases.

Chronic and progressive anaemia are major problems associated with malaria, especially in children and pregnant women. In cases where the oxygen content of the blood is reduced beyond a critical point, blood transfusions may be needed. Of course this presents major problems in areas where blood is not routinely screened for HIV, or is not available.

Tourists and travellers to malaria endemic areas are advised to know their blood group, and if possible draw up a list of potential blood donors with whom they are familiar, and whom they can trust not to have AIDS.

Table 7: Information required by doctor before treatment

❖ Which species of malaria parasite is prevalent in country of destination?
[ ] falciparum   [ ] vivax   [ ] malariae   [ ] ovale

❖ Which drug was used for chemoprophylaxis during visit?

❖ When did you first start taking the chemoprophylaxis?
Date:_____

❖ When did you stop taking the chemoprophylaxis?
Date:_____

❖ How often was it taken?
[ ] once a week   [ ] daily   [ ] other_____

❖ Did you take it conscientiously and at about the same time every day or week?

❖ At what dosage was the drug taken?
[ ] one tablet   [ ] two tablets   [ ] other_____

❖ Is there any aspect of your medical history that should be noted by a doctor prescribing drugs for the treatment of malaria?
[ ] pregnancy   [ ] hypoglycaemia   [ ] hepatitis
[ ] kidney disorder   [ ] sulfa sensitivity
[ ] cardiac condition [ ] depressive condition
[ ] other_____

Table 8: Information necessary for prescribing antimalarials to travellers

---

✧ Which species of malaria parasite is prevalent in country of destination?

[ ] falciparum   [ ] vivax   [ ] malariae   [ ] ovale

✧ Drug sensitivity list: Which drugs work best for treatment in country of destination?

✧ Is there any aspect of your medical history that should be noted by a doctor prescribing drugs for the prevention of malaria?

[ ] pregnancy   [ ] hypoglycaemia   [ ] hepatitis
[ ] kidney disorder   [ ] sulfa sensitivity
[ ] cardiac condition [ ] depressive condition
[ ] other _____

Appendix 2: Prophylaxis

Warning

Remember that no drug is 100 per cent effective. Even though you may comply with drug dosage instructions, you may still contract malaria. Drug prophylaxis remains controversial and recommendations are constantly changing.

Chemoprophylaxis and stand-by medicament

The following summarises the situation when chemoprophylaxis and stand-by treatment may be considered; detailed recommendations are given in *International Travel and Health — Vaccination Requirements and Health Advice* (published by the WHO).

Chemoprophylaxis and stand-by medicament are not recommended in areas where transmission of malaria has not been reported or occurs only at a very low level, and where suitable diagnostic and therapeutic facilities are within easy reach.

Chemoprophylaxis is not recommended but stand-by medicament is to be available in areas where transmission of malaria is low and diagnostic and therapeutic facilities are not readily available.

Chemoprophylaxis is recommended but stand-by medicament is not required in areas where chemoprophylaxis would be expected to be successful. These are areas with chloroquine-sensitive *P. falciparum* and areas with *P. vivax*, *P. malariae* or both but without *P. falciparum*. Chloroquine is the prophylactic of choice but an alternative drug needs to be carried.

Both chemoprophylaxis and stand-by medicament are recommended for travellers to areas where a reasonable risk of infection with *P. falciparum* exists, and where the drug used for prophylaxis may not be effective in preventing clinical illness.

If adequate measures for personal protection can be ensured, it may be acceptable to rely on these methods without any chemoprophylaxis but with an appropriate stand-by drug.

Different options of chemoprophylaxis with or without stand-by medicament are available. If adequate measures for personal protection can be ensured, it may be sufficient to rely on these methods without any chemoprophylaxis but with an appropriate stand-by drug.

In the event of illness, it is vital for travellers to obtain treatment from a qualified medical practitioner.

In the past, it was thought that malaria chemoprophylaxis in non-immune people was of benefit and without serious complications and that, consequently, it was better for travellers to take prophylaxis if their risk of acquiring malaria was uncertain.

Drugs for prophylaxis and treatment (see also page 91)

Compound	Trade names
Chloroquine-phosphate:	Aralen, Avloclor, Delagil, Lagaquin, Lariago, Malaviron, Resochin, Starquine
Chloroquine-sulph:	Nivaquine
Hydroxychloroquine-sulph:	Plaguenil (not often used for malaria, more for rheumatoid arthritis)
Mefloquine:	Mephaquin, Lariam

Drugs for prophylaxis only

Compound	Trade names
Doxycycline:	Vibramycin
Dapsone-pyrimethamine:	Maloprim
Proguanil:	Paludrine, Paludrinol
Pyrimethamine:	Daraprim, Tindurin
Sulphametopyrazine-pyrimethamine:	Metakelfin
Chlorproguanil:	Lapudrine
Chloroquine-pyrimethamine:	Daraclor

Chloroquine

Chloroquine has been the most relied upon prophylactic for many years. Taken widely, it has, to its own detriment, helped to create widespread resistance to its prophylactic powers (see chloroquine resistance, page 93). Despite this there are still areas where chloroquine is useful as a prophylactic, especially in combination with proguanil (Paludrine). (See also contra-indications and side effects of chloroquine, page 94.)

Chloroquine-pyrimethamine (Daraclor)

Daraclor has a chloroquine base and has a similar effect to chloroquine although it is used only for prophylaxis. The combination is thought to confer only marginal benefit over the use of chloroquine alone. If taken during pregnancy, a folic acid supplement must be used.

Side effects include headache, gastrointestinal disturbances such as nausea and vomiting, diarrhoea and abdominal cramps, pruritus and macular, urticarial and purpuric skin eruptions. Patients with liver or kidney problems or porphyria and psoriasis should take special care when taking Daraclor.

Dapsone-pyrimethamine (Maloprim)

Used as a prophylactic and not as a treatment. Serious side effects occur only if the recommended dose is exceeded. These include folic acid deficiency, agranulocytosis, anaemia. Its efficacy as a prophylactic has been questioned.

The use of Maloprim during the third trimester of pregnancy should be avoided and if taken during the first and second trimesters, a folic acid supplement is recommended.

For **Mefloquine** see page 98.

Pyrimethamine (Daraprim)

Used as a prophylactic and not as a treatment. However, the use of this drug on its own is not recommended as it is slow acting and numerous breakthroughs by *P. falciparum* have been reported in southern Africa.

Proguanil (Paludrine)

Formerly taken on its own, proguanil has been taken safely for over 40 years. Its use is now recommended in combination with chloroquine even in areas where chloroquine resistance exists, as it appears to give greater protection in this combination than when used alone.

Proguanil can safely be used during pregnancy and for children and rarely causes side effects. Those most frequently reported are mouth ulcers, hair loss, vomiting and abdominal discomfort. It is thought but not proven that a folic acid supplement may help ameliorate these side effects.

Doxycycline (Vibramycin)

This is a useful alternative when mefloquine or proguanil is unavailable or contra-indicated in areas with chloroquine-resistant malaria. Its use is recommended for short-term travellers only (less than eight weeks).

Doxycycline is contra-indicated in pregnant and breastfeeding women and in children under the age of eight.

The most common side effects include gastrointestinal disturbances such as nausea and diarrhoea; sensitivity to light characterised by exaggerated sunburn, a number of dermatological reactions and vaginal thrush.

Bibliography

Cahill, Kevin M. and William O'Brien. *Tropical medicine — a clinical text.* Heinemann Medical Books, London, 1990

Fripp, Peter J. *An introduction to human parasitology with reference to southern Africa.* 2nd edition. Macmillan South Africa, Johannesburg, 1983

Guidelines for the diagnosis and treatment of malaria in Africa. Afro Technical Papers No 22. Report of an informal consultation of experts on malaria in the African region. World Health Organization Regional Office for Africa, Brazzaville, 1990

IATA. *Travel information manual.* International Air Traffic Association, Amsterdam, 1993

Manson-Bahr, P.E.C. *Manson's tropical diseases.* 19th edition. Bailliere-Tindall, London, 1987.

Ransford, Oliver. *Bid the sickness cease — disease in the history of Black Africa.* John Murray, London, 1983

South Africa, Department of National Health and Population Development. *Malaria prophylaxis — the South African viewpoint.* Government Printer, Pretoria, 1992

The South African Medical Journal, February/March 1993

Targett, G.A.T. (ed.) *Malaria — waiting for the vaccine.* John Wiley & Sons, London, 1991

WHO. *International travel and health — vaccination requirements and health advice,* World Health Organization, Geneva, 1992

WHO Scientific Group. *Practical chemotherapy of malaria.* Technical Report Series, No. 805, World Health Organization, Geneva, 1990

Index